GW01459386

The Power of Breath

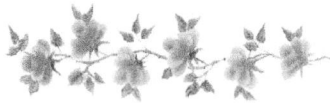

A Comprehensive Guide to
Mastering 21 Breathing Techniques
for Health, Focus, and Well-Being

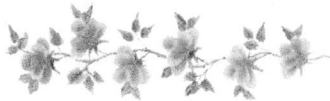

Melody Wallack

ISBN: 9798393817596

Imprint: Independently published

Cover design by: Echo Enterprise LLC.

Library of Congress Control Number: 2018675309

Printed in the United States of America

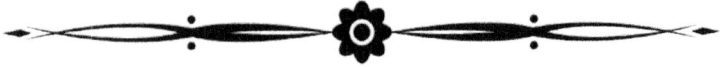

DISCLAIMER

The information provided in this book is intended for educational and informational purposes only. It should not be used as a substitute for professional medical advice, diagnosis, or treatment. The author and publisher do not provide any kind of professional advice, including medical or psychological advice. It is important to consult with a qualified healthcare provider or professional for any specific health questions or concerns.

The techniques and strategies presented in this book may not be effective for everyone, as individual circumstances and experiences can vary. The author and publisher make no guarantees or promises regarding any specific outcomes or results from using the information presented in this book.

If you require professional medical, legal, financial, or mental health advice or treatment, please seek out the appropriate qualified professionals. The author and publisher of this book are not responsible for any adverse effects or consequences resulting from the use or application of the information contained in this book.

By purchasing or reading this book, you agree to hold harmless the author, publisher, and any other associated parties from any liability arising from errors, omissions, inaccuracies, or misrepresentations in the content. It is also important to acknowledge that web-linked content may change over time, and certain events may have been modified. The author and publisher offer no guarantees or warranties in relation to the information provided within the book.

The reader assumes full responsibility for any actions taken based on the information contained in this book. The author and publisher of this book are not responsible for any loss, damage, or injury caused or alleged to be caused, directly or indirectly, by the information presented herein.

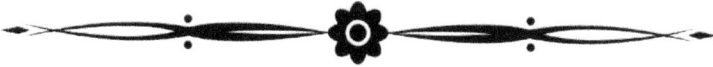

TABLE OF CONTENTS

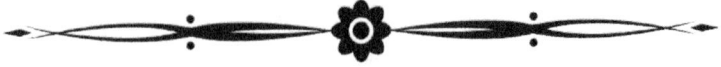

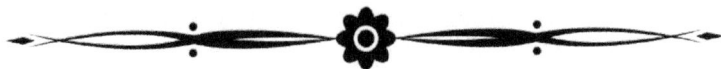

INTRODUCTION

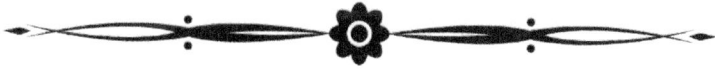

Breath is the essence of life. It is the first thing we do when we are born, and the last thing we do before we leave this world. Despite its fundamental importance, many of us rarely give our breath the attention it deserves. As a naturopathy doctor (ND) in training, a meditator for more than 30 years, and a lifelong enthusiast of health, nutrition, and fitness, I have come to understand the profound impact that conscious breathing can have on our overall well-being.

Throughout my journey, I have explored various natural modalities to improve the body's balance and harmony, such as herbology, nutrition, ozone therapy, Bach Flowers, sound, and many more modalities. Among these practices, I have found breathing techniques to be one of the most accessible, powerful, affordable, and transformative tools available to us. With over 30 years of meditation experience, I have discovered a wealth of breathing techniques that can positively influence our mental, emotional, and physical states.

This book, "*The Power of Breath*," is a culmination of my passion for sharing the knowledge and wisdom I have gained throughout my life and my studies in naturopathy. It is designed to be a comprehensive guide to mastering various breathing techniques for enhancing health, focus, and well-being. The techniques outlined in this book cater to a diverse range of needs and preferences, from relaxation and stress relief to energy and focus, as well as specific conditions that can benefit from targeted breathwork.

My goal in writing this book is to provide you with a solid understanding of the anatomy and physiology of the respiratory system, the connection between breath and mental/emotional states, and the benefits of practicing conscious breathing. You will learn 21 different breathing techniques, each with detailed instructions, benefits, and precautions. Additionally, this book will guide you in *combining and customizing these techniques to create a personalized daily breathing practice tailored to your unique needs and goals.*

Breathing is a fundamental aspect of life, yet it's something that many of us take for granted. We often overlook the power that lies within each breath we take and its potential to significantly impact our overall well-being. In this book, we will explore:

a. **Importance of proper breathing**: The way we breathe directly affects our physical, mental, and emotional health. Proper breathing is crucial for maintaining balance in our autonomic nervous system, supporting the optimal function of our organs, and ensuring mental clarity. Improper breathing can contribute to various health issues, such as stress, anxiety, and sleep disturbances. By understanding the mechanics and significance of proper breathing, we can take steps to improve our well-being.

b. **Benefits of practicing breathing techniques**: Incorporating breathing techniques into our daily lives offers numerous benefits. These practices can promote relaxation, stress reduction, increased energy, improved focus, and enhanced emotional well-being. Moreover, specific techniques can support the management of health conditions such as asthma, anxiety, and chronic pain. By exploring and practicing various breathing techniques, we can harness the power of our breath to improve our overall quality of life.

c. **Overview of the various techniques included in the book**: This comprehensive guide covers 21 different breathing techniques, each with its unique set of benefits and applications. The techniques are categorized based on their primary purposes, such as relaxation and stress relief, energy and focus, balance and mindfulness, and addressing specific conditions. The book provides detailed instructions, benefits, and precautions for each technique, as well as guidance on combining and customizing techniques to meet individual needs and preferences. Additionally, readers will find valuable resources for further exploration and practice.

By embarking on this journey of breath exploration, I hope you will come to appreciate the profound power that lies within each inhalation and exhalation. You will uncover the remarkable potential of conscious breathing to enhance your health, focus, and well-being. This book aims to serve as a valuable resource and companion in your quest to harness the transformative power of the breath. May this book serve as a valuable resource and companion on your path to greater health, focus, and well-being through the art of conscious breathing.

With "*The Power of Breath*," you will be equipped with the knowledge, tools, and techniques to embark on a life-changing journey towards better health and a more balanced, harmonious life. As you delve into the world of conscious breathing, you will uncover the hidden potential within each breath, empowering you to take control of your well-being and unlock the full range of benefits that proper breathing has to offer.

As you progress through this book and experiment with the various techniques, remember that the key to success lies in consistency and commitment. Find the techniques that resonate with you and practice them regularly to see the true impact of conscious breathing on your life. In time, you may discover that the simple act of breathing has the power to transform not only your physical health but also your mental and emotional well-being, paving the way for a more balanced, fulfilled, and vibrant life.

Embrace the journey, and remember that with every breath you take, you hold the key to unlocking your full potential. Here's to your journey towards greater health, focus, and well-being through the transformative power of the breath.

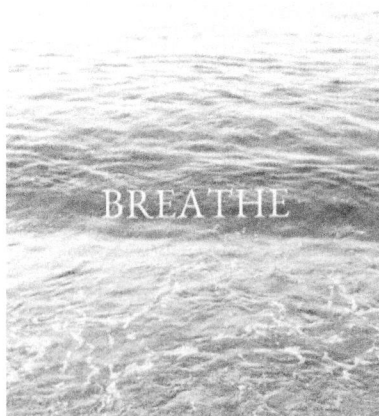

Chapter 1

The Vital Importance of Breathing

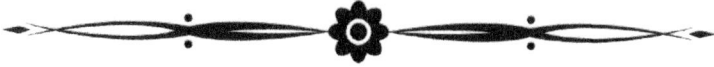

Breathing is vital for life. It's a question that may seem silly at first glance - why do we have to breathe? But the truth is, without breath, we cannot survive. This fact is illustrated in emergency situations, like the one a young girl named Lilly experiences when she calls 911 for her unconscious mother. In that moment, Lilly is coached through CPR and instructed to check her mother's breathing.

Ring ring…

911 Operator: "911, what's your emergency?"

Lilly: "My mom just collapsed, and she won't wake up. I don't know what to do!"

911 Operator: "I understand, ma'am. Please remain calm and tell me your location so we can send help right away."

Lilly: "We're at 3465 Washington Avenue."

911 Operator: "Okay, help is on the way. Is your mom breathing?"

Lilly: "I don't know, I haven't checked."

911 Operator: "It's important to check her breathing right now. Can you do that for me?"

Lilly: "Okay, hold on."

(Short pause)

Lilly: "I can't tell if she's breathing or not!"

911 Operator: "That's okay, I'm going to guide you through it. Listen carefully and follow my instructions. First, place your ear close to her mouth and nose to see if you can feel or hear any breath. Can you tell me what you hear or feel?"

Lilly: "I can feel some air coming out of her nose."

911 Operator: "Good job, now we need to start CPR right away. Do you know how to do CPR?"

Lilly: "I learned it in my health class, but I'm not sure if I can do it right!"

911 Operator: "Don't worry, I'll talk you through it step by step. We need to act quickly to help your mom. Put one hand on top of the other and place them in the center of her chest. Push down hard and fast, like this: one, two, three, four. Keep going until the ambulance arrives. Can you do that for me?"

Lilly: "Yes, I can do that."

911 Operator: "Great, keep going and stay on the line with me until the ambulance arrives. You're doing a great job, Lilly. Your mom is lucky to have you."

This scenario may seem familiar, whether from personal experience or depictions in movies or TV shows. And in the age of COVID-19, we've seen countless patients being intubated in hospitals to artificially help them breathe. It's clear that breath is a vital component of life. In fact, respiratory rate is one of the vital signs doctors and nurses check when monitoring our health.

Consider the *rule of three: humans can survive three weeks without food, three days without water, but only three minutes without breathing.* With this in mind, it's clear that breath is an essential aspect of our existence.

In this book, we'll explore 21 different breathing techniques, each with its own unique benefits. These include techniques like diaphragmatic breathing, Zen breathing, relaxing breathing, and more.

But before we dive into these techniques, it's important to understand the basics of breathing. How does it work? What happens when we breathe in versus when we breathe out? In the following sections, we'll explore the essentials of breathing before exploring the intricacies of each technique.

It's understandable that reading about emergency situations like Lilly's may cause anxiety or fear. However, the purpose of sharing this story is not to cause distress, but rather to emphasize the importance of breathing for our survival. Whether we are facing a medical emergency or simply going about our daily lives, breathing is a vital and often overlooked aspect of our health and wellbeing.

With the knowledge and techniques shared in this book, we can take control of our breath and improve our physical, mental, and emotional health. So, take a deep breath and let's begin our journey towards the power of breathing.

Chapter 2

Understanding the Basics of Breathing

1. **Anatomy of the Respiratory System**
   a) **The Nose and Nasal Cavity**: The nose and nasal cavity are the primary entry points for air into the respiratory system. The nasal cavity filters, warms, and

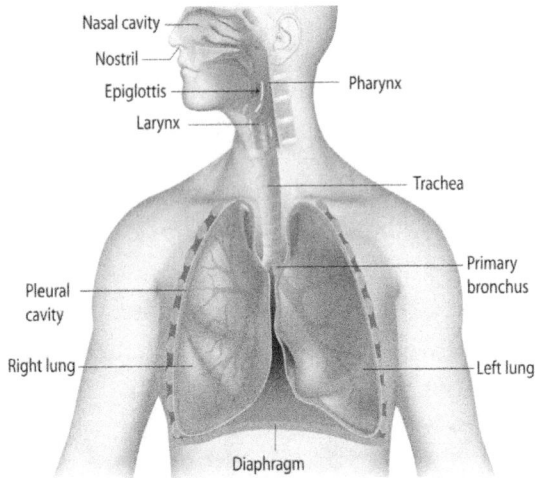

humidifies the incoming air to prepare it for the lungs. Tiny hair-like structures called cilia and a layer of mucus help trap dust, allergens, and other particles.
   b) **The Mouth and Oral Cavity**: The mouth is an alternative entry point for air, especially during times of increased oxygen demand, such as during exercise. While the mouth doesn't filter air as

efficiently as the nasal cavity, it does allow for a greater volume of air to enter the respiratory system.

c) **The Pharynx and Larynx:** The pharynx, or throat, is a muscular tube that connects the nasal and oral cavities to the larynx (voice box). The larynx houses the vocal cords and helps protect the trachea from foreign objects by closing the epiglottis, a flap of cartilage, during swallowing.

d) **The Trachea, Bronchi, and Bronchioles**: The trachea, or windpipe, is a tube that carries air from the larynx to the bronchi, which are the two main

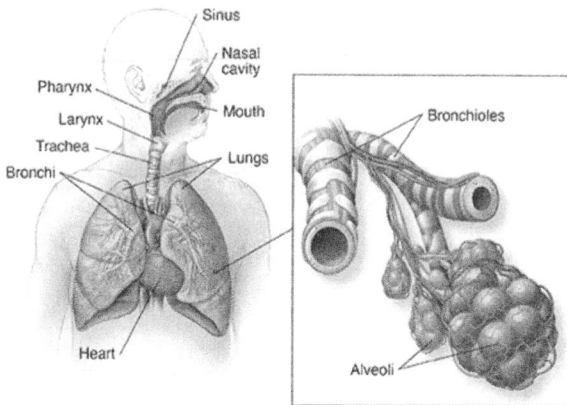

branches that connect to each lung. The bronchi further divide into smaller tubes called bronchioles, which eventually lead to the alveoli.

e) **The Lungs and Alveoli**: The lungs are a pair of spongy, elastic organs responsible for gas exchange. Within the lungs, there are millions of tiny air sacs called alveoli, where oxygen from the inhaled air diffuses into the bloodstream, and carbon dioxide from the blood is expelled through exhalation.

f) **The Diaphragm and Intercostal Muscles**: The diaphragm is a dome-shaped muscle located below the lungs that plays a vital role in breathing. During inhalation, the diaphragm contracts and moves downward, increasing the volume of the chest cavity and allowing the lungs to expand. The intercostal muscles, located between the ribs, also assist in the expansion and contraction of the ribcage during breathing.

2. **Physiology of Breathing**
   a) **Inhalation and Exhalation**: Inhalation is the process of drawing air into the lungs, while exhalation is the release of air from the lungs. Both processes result from changes in the pressure within the chest cavity, which is regulated by the contraction and relaxation of the diaphragm and intercostal muscles.

   b) **Gas Exchange in the Lungs**: Gas exchange occurs within the alveoli, where oxygen from inhaled air diffuses into the surrounding capillaries and binds to hemoglobin molecules in red blood cells. Simultaneously, carbon dioxide, a waste product from cellular respiration, diffuses from the blood into the alveoli and is expelled during exhalation.

   c) **Oxygen Transport in the Blood**: Oxygen bound to hemoglobin is transported through the bloodstream to cells and tissues throughout the body, where it is released and used for cellular respiration. The oxygen-depleted blood then returns to the lungs to be reoxygenated.

d) **The Role of Carbon Dioxide in Breathing**: Carbon dioxide plays a crucial role in regulating breathing. High levels of carbon dioxide in the blood stimulate the respiratory center in the brain, increasing the rate and depth of breathing to help expel the excess carbon dioxide.

e) **The Respiratory Center and Control of Breathing**: The respiratory center, located in the medulla oblongata of the brain, controls the rate and depth of breathing by sending signals to the diaphragm and intercostal muscles. The respiratory center receives input from various sources, including chemoreceptors that detect levels of oxygen, carbon dioxide, and pH in the blood, as well as input from the higher brain centers related to emotions, pain, and voluntary control of breathing.

3. **The Connection between Breath, Mind, and Emotions**
   a) **The Autonomic Nervous System**: The autonomic nervous system (ANS) is a part of the nervous system that regulates involuntary functions, such as heart rate, digestion, and breathing. The ANS is divided into two branches: the sympathetic nervous system, which is responsible for the "fight or flight" response and increases arousal, and the parasympathetic nervous system, which is responsible for the "rest and digest" response and promotes relaxation.

   b) **The Stress Response and the Relaxation Response**: The way we breathe can directly influence our stress response and relaxation response. Rapid, shallow breathing is associated with the activation of the sympathetic nervous system, while slow, deep breathing activates the parasympathetic nervous system, promoting relaxation and stress reduction.

c) **Breath and Emotional Regulation**: Breathing practices can help regulate emotions by influencing the ANS and altering the balance between the sympathetic and parasympathetic nervous systems. Conscious control of breathing can provide a means to self-regulate emotions, reduce anxiety, and increase feelings of calm and well-being.

d) **Breath and Mental Focus:** Focused breathing practices, such as meditation and mindfulness, can improve mental focus and clarity by increasing awareness of the present moment and reducing the effects of stress and anxiety on cognitive function.

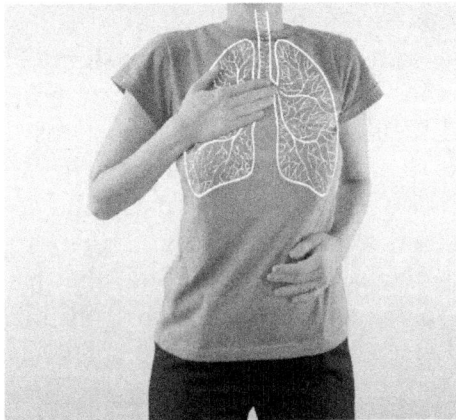

Chapter 3

21 Breathing Techniques in Detail

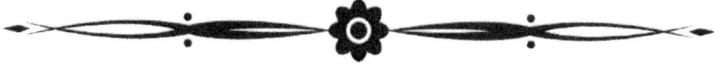

Unlock the Power of Breathing with These 21 Techniques for Improved Health and Well-being.

In this chapter, we will explore 21 different breathing techniques, each with its own unique benefits. Building on the basics of breathing covered in the previous chapter, we will dive into the intricacies of each technique, including their history, specific benefits, variations and techniques, case studies or personal anecdotes, scientific research and studies, cultural and spiritual origins, practical tips and exercises for daily practice, precautions, and contraindications, as well as further resources and recommendations.

Whether you're looking to reduce stress and anxiety, improve your lung function, or simply enhance your overall well-being, these techniques offer a range of tools for taking control of your breath and improving your physical, mental, and emotional health.

It's worth noting that some of these techniques may overlap or be similar to other breathing methods. However, the purpose of this chapter is to provide you with a comprehensive guide to each technique, so that you can fully understand and practice each one individually. Whether you are a beginner or an experienced breathwork practitioner, this chapter offers valuable information and guidance for exploring the vast world of breathing techniques. So, feel free to pick and choose the techniques that resonate with you and incorporate them into your daily routine.

1. **Diaphragmatic Breathing**

    History and Origins: Diaphragmatic breathing, also known as belly breathing or abdominal breathing, has roots in traditional yogic breathing techniques. The practice of diaphragmatic breathing has been used in various cultures and traditions, including Chinese medicine and martial arts, for centuries.

    Specific Benefits: Diaphragmatic breathing can help reduce stress and anxiety, lower blood pressure, improve lung function, and promote relaxation. It can also help individuals with chronic obstructive pulmonary disease (COPD), asthma, and other respiratory conditions.

    Variations and Techniques: Diaphragmatic breathing involves the contraction and relaxation of the diaphragm muscle, which is located below the lungs.

    Step-by-step guide on how to practice diaphragmatic breathing:

    1. Find a comfortable position: You can either lie on your back or sit upright in a chair with your back straight. Ensure that you're comfortable and relaxed.

    2. Place your hands on your belly and chest: Place one hand on your belly and the other on your chest. This will help you become more aware of your breathing.

3. Inhale deeply through your nose: Take a slow, deep breath through your nose. As you inhale, focus on filling your lungs with air and feel your belly expand outward. Ensure that your chest remains relatively still as you breathe.

4. Exhale through your mouth: Slowly exhale through your mouth while contracting your diaphragm muscles. You should feel your belly fall inward as you exhale.

5. Repeat: Repeat this process for 5-10 minutes, focusing on your breath and the movement of your belly.

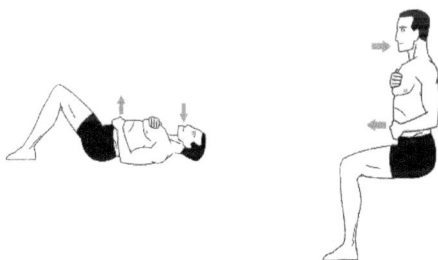

Case Studies or Personal Anecdotes: Many individuals have reported benefits from practicing diaphragmatic breathing, including improved relaxation, better sleep, and reduced stress and anxiety.

Scientific Research and Studies: Numerous studies have shown the effectiveness of diaphragmatic breathing for reducing stress, anxiety, and blood pressure. One study found that practicing diaphragmatic breathing for 20 minutes a day for eight weeks significantly reduced systolic and diastolic blood pressure in hypertensive patients. Another study found that practicing diaphragmatic breathing improved the lung function of individuals with COPD.

Cultural and Spiritual Origins: Diaphragmatic breathing has roots in traditional yogic breathing techniques and is a key component of pranayama practices.

Practical Tips and Exercises for Daily Practice: To incorporate diaphragmatic breathing into daily life, individuals can practice for a few minutes each day, gradually increasing the duration over time. It is best to practice diaphragmatic breathing in a quiet and comfortable space, free from distractions.

Precautions and Contraindications: Individuals with certain medical conditions, such as hernias or hiatal hernias, should consult with their healthcare provider before practicing diaphragmatic breathing.

Further Resources and Recommendations: Additional resources for learning and practicing diaphragmatic breathing include online tutorials, books on breathing techniques, and guided meditation apps.

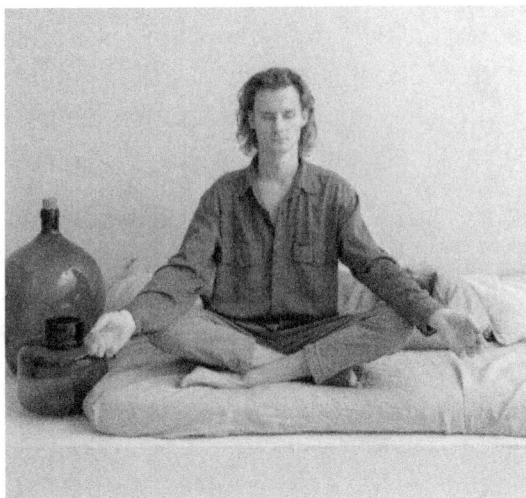

Diaphragmatic breathing

By Melody Wallack

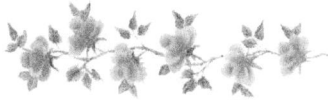

Inhale and let your belly expand,

Exhale and feel the tension disband,

Breathe deep, slow and controlled,

Let your diaphragm be your stronghold.

***

Stress and anxiety have no place,

When you breathe with such grace,

Relaxation and peace is what you'll find,

Through diaphragmatic breathing, you'll unwind.

***

Your breath is the key to your soul,

It can bring you to a place that's whole,

So let each inhale and exhale be,

A mindful moment, just for thee.

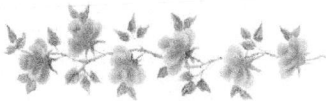

2. Zen Breathing:

Zen breathing, also known as Zazen breathing or Hara breathing, is a breathing technique that originated in Zen Buddhism as part of meditation practice. The technique involves slow, deep breathing focused on the lower abdomen or hara, a term in Japanese culture that refers to the center of physical and spiritual energy.

History and Origins: Zen breathing has its roots in the practice of Zazen, a form of seated meditation that has been part of Zen Buddhism for centuries. In Zazen, practitioners focus on their breath as a means of achieving mindfulness and awareness of the present moment.

Specific Benefits: Zen breathing has been shown to have numerous benefits, including reducing stress and anxiety, improving cognitive function and mental clarity, and promoting relaxation and well-being.

Variations and Techniques: Zen breathing involves slow, deep breaths through the nose, focusing on the lower abdomen or hara. The exhale should be longer than the inhale, and the breath should be smooth and continuous. The goal of the practice is to cultivate a sense of calm and awareness, while also developing strength in the lower abdominal muscles.

Step-by-step format for Zen Breathing:

1. Find a comfortable seated position, with your back straight and your hands resting on your thighs.

2. Close your eyes and take a few deep breaths through your nose, letting your breath flow naturally.

3. Begin to focus your attention on your lower abdomen, imagining the breath moving in and out of this area.

4. Inhale slowly and deeply through your nose, feeling your belly expand with the breath.

5. Exhale slowly through your nose, feeling your belly contract and drawing the breath out as long as possible.

6. Repeat this slow, deep breathing pattern, focusing on the sensation of the breath moving in and out of your lower abdomen.

7. If your mind begins to wander, gently bring your attention back to your breath and the movement of your lower abdomen.

8. Continue the practice for several minutes, gradually extending the length of your exhale to become longer than your inhale.

9. When you are ready to end the practice, take a few more deep breaths, feeling a sense of calm and awareness in your body and mind.

Recommended duration: 5-10 minutes.

Case Studies or Personal Anecdotes: Many individuals have reported experiencing a greater sense of calm and clarity after practicing Zen breathing. Some have also reported improved sleep and reduced symptoms of anxiety and depression.

Scientific Research and Studies: Studies have shown that deep breathing techniques, including Zen breathing, can help reduce stress and anxiety by activating the parasympathetic nervous system and decreasing the activity of the sympathetic nervous system. Additionally, research has found that deep breathing can improve cognitive function and decrease symptoms of depression.

Cultural and Spiritual Origins: Zen breathing has its roots in Zen Buddhism, which emphasizes the practice of mindfulness and awareness in daily life. The technique is often used as a means of developing greater focus and clarity in meditation practice.

Practical Tips and Exercises for Daily Practice: To practice Zen breathing, find a comfortable seated position and focus on your breath, directing it toward your lower abdomen. Inhale slowly through your nose, feeling your belly expand. Exhale slowly through your nose, feeling your belly contract. Aim for a slow and steady breath, keeping your mind focused on the sensation of the breath moving in and out of your body.

Precautions and Contraindications: Zen breathing is generally safe for most individuals to practice, but those with certain medical conditions, such as asthma or chronic obstructive pulmonary disease (COPD), should consult a healthcare provider before starting a new breathing practice.

Further Resources and Recommendations: Books on Zen meditation and breathing techniques, such as "Zen Mind, Beginner's Mind" by Shunryu Suzuki and "The Art of Just Sitting: Essential Writings on the Zen Practice of Shikantaza" by John Daido Loori, can provide further guidance on the practice of Zen breathing. Additionally, attending a meditation class or workshop with a qualified instructor can be helpful in developing a regular practice.

Zen Breathing

By Melody Wallack

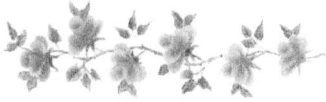

Inhale, exhale, the breath is still
The mind is calm, the body's will
To move, to act, to be at peace
All can be found within release
***

The breath is deep, the chest expands
The air flows in, like waves on sand
The body still, the mind serene
In this moment, all can be seen
***

With each exhale, the tension's gone
The worries fade, like morning's dawn
The breath is life, the breath is free
In Zen breathing, we find our key.

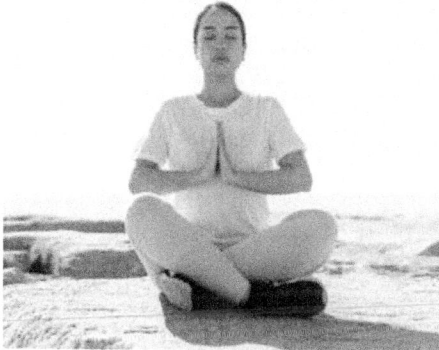

3. Relaxing Breathing (4-7-8 Breathing)

History and Origins: Relaxing breathing, also known as 4-7-8 breathing, was developed by Dr. Andrew Weil, an American physician and author, as a simple and effective way to reduce stress and anxiety.

Specific Benefits: 4-7-8 breathing has been shown to be effective in reducing stress and anxiety, lowering blood pressure, and improving sleep quality. It can also be helpful for managing anger and reducing cravings.

Variations and Techniques: Step by step for 4-7-8 breathing technique:

1. Find a comfortable seated position with your back straight and your feet flat on the ground.

2. Close your mouth and place the tip of your tongue behind your upper front teeth, keeping it there throughout the exercise.

3. Inhale slowly and deeply through your nose for a count of four.

4. Hold your breath for a count of seven.

5. Exhale slowly and completely through your mouth, making a *whooshing sound*, for a count of eight.

6. This completes one round of the technique. Repeat the cycle three more times, for a total of four rounds.

7. After the final round, sit quietly for a few moments and observe how you feel.

Case Studies or Personal Anecdotes: Many individuals have reported experiencing significant reductions in stress and anxiety after incorporating 4-7-8 breathing into their daily routine. Some have also reported improved sleep quality and better ability to manage anger and cravings.

Scientific Research and Studies: A study published in the Journal of Medical Science and Clinical Research found that practicing 4-7-8 breathing for eight weeks significantly reduced anxiety levels in participants. Another study published in the International Journal of Behavioral Medicine found that the technique improved sleep quality and reduced symptoms of insomnia in participants.

Cultural and Spiritual Origins: While 4-7-8 breathing was developed in a Western medical context, it draws on principles from traditional Eastern practices such as yoga and meditation, which have long emphasized the connection between breath, mind, and body.

Practical Tips and Exercises for Daily Practice: Incorporating 4-7-8 breathing into your daily routine can be as simple as taking a few minutes to practice the technique when you wake up or before going to bed. You can also use it throughout the day as a tool for managing stress and anxiety.

Precautions and Contraindications: As with any breathing technique, it is important to listen to your body and not push yourself beyond your limits. If you experience dizziness or lightheadedness while practicing 4-7-8 breathing, stop the exercise and return to normal breathing.

Further Resources and Recommendations: For more information on 4-7-8 breathing and how to incorporate it into your daily routine, Dr. Andrew Weil's website provides a detailed guide to the technique, as well as additional resources and tips for managing stress and anxiety.

Relaxing Breathing (4-7-8 Breathing)

By Melody Wallack

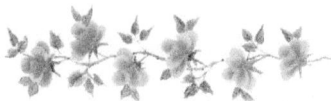

Inhale deeply, count to four,
Hold the breath, count to seven more.
Exhale slowly, count to eight,
Release the tension, feel the weight.

***

Relaxing breathing, a simple tool,
To calm the mind and body cool.
With every breath, the stress departs,
The mind grows still, the soul restarts.

***

Inhale peace, hold joy inside,
Exhale worries, let them subside.
With each breath, find the calm,
A peaceful state, a soothing balm.

***

Relaxing breathing, a gift to give,
A way to live, a way to live.

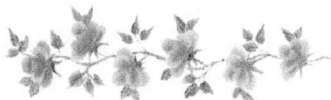

4.Stimulating Breathing (Bellows breath (Bhastrika))

History and Origins: Bellows breath, also known as Bhastrika, is an ancient yogic breathing technique that originates from India. The term "Bhastrika" is derived from the Sanskrit word "bhastrika," which means "bellows." This technique has been practiced for centuries as a way to energize the body and mind. This technique involves rapid, forceful inhalations and exhalations, similar to the way a blacksmith bellows works. It is known to help energize the body, improve lung capacity, and stimulate the nervous system.

Specific Benefits: Bellows breath is known for its ability to invigorate the body and mind. It can increase oxygenation and blood flow, providing a burst of energy and mental clarity. It may also help to relieve stress, anxiety, and depression.

Variations and Techniques:

Bellows breath involves rapid and forceful inhalations and exhalations through the nose, similar to the movement of bellows. The technique can be performed in different variations, including slow and steady, or rapid and forceful, depending on the practitioner's preference.

Step-by-step instructions for practicing Bellows Breath:

1. Sit comfortably with your spine straight and your hands resting on your knees.

2. Take a few deep breaths through your nose to prepare.

3. Inhale deeply through your nose and then forcefully exhale out through your nose.

4. Inhale forcefully through your nose and then forcefully exhale out through your nose.

5. Continue this rapid, forceful pattern for up to one minute, taking short breaks if needed.

6. After one minute, take a few deep breaths to return to your normal breathing pattern.

7. You can repeat this exercise for up to five minutes.

It's important to note that Bellows Breath can be intense and may not be suitable for everyone, especially those with respiratory problems or high blood pressure. It's best to practice under the guidance of a qualified practitioner and to listen to your body's signals during the exercise.

Case Studies or Personal Anecdotes: One individual reported experiencing significant improvements in their energy levels and focus after incorporating bellows breath into their daily routine. Another individual found that regular practice of this technique helped them to manage symptoms of anxiety and stress.

Scientific Research and Studies: Limited scientific research has been conducted on the specific effects of bellows breath. However, studies have suggested that yogic breathing practices, in general, can help to reduce stress and improve mental well-being.

Cultural and Spiritual Origins: Bellows breath is an ancient yogic breathing technique that has been practiced in India for centuries as a way to stimulate the body and mind.

Practical Tips and Exercises for Daily Practice: Bellows breath can be practiced for one to three minutes at a time, depending on the practitioner's level of comfort. It is important to start slowly and gradually increase the pace and intensity of the breath.

Precautions and Contraindications: Bellows breath may not be suitable for individuals with certain medical conditions, such as hypertension, cardiovascular disease, or glaucoma. It is important to consult with a healthcare professional before beginning any new breathing practice.

Further Resources and Recommendations: For more information on bellows breath and other yogic breathing techniques, readers may refer to the following resources:

1. "The Science of Pranayama" by Sri Swami Sivananda

2. "The Yoga of Breath: A Step-by-Step Guide to Pranayama" by Richard Rosen

3. Online resources and classes on yogic breathing techniques, such as those offered by the Yoga Alliance.

Stimulating breathing (Bellows breath)

By Melody Wallack

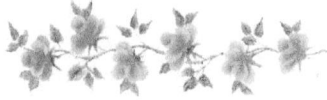

Inhale, exhale, fire in the belly,

Bellows breath ignites energy so steady,

Rhythmic pumping, chest rising high,

Prana flowing, spirit soaring to the sky.

***

Stimulating breath, oh mighty power,

Igniting life force in every hour,

With each breath, a spark of light,

Leading to a path of pure delight.

***

Breath in, breath out, with each beat of the heart,

Bellows breath, a practice that sets us apart,

A tool for transformation, a key to the soul,

Let the fire within you burn and make you whole.

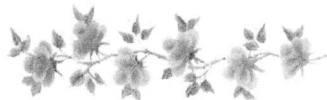

5. Anchoring Breathing

Anchoring Breathing is a technique that combines deep breathing with visualization or a mantra to help anchor the mind. This practice is designed to help individuals stay grounded and focused, particularly during times of stress or anxiety.

History and origins: The origins of Anchoring Breathing are not well-documented, but the technique has become increasingly popular in recent years as a tool for managing stress and improving mental clarity.

Specific benefits: Anchoring Breathing has been shown to have a variety of benefits for mental and emotional well-being. By combining deep breathing with visualization or a physical anchor, this practice can help reduce stress and anxiety, improve focus and concentration, and promote a sense of calm and inner peace.

Variations and techniques: Anchoring Breathing can be practiced in various ways, depending on personal preferences and individual needs. Some people prefer to focus on a particular image or phrase during the practice, while others may use a physical anchor such as a crystal or piece of jewelry.

As you continue to breathe deeply, visualize your chosen image or phrase in your mind's eye, or focus on the physical sensation of your anchor. With each inhale, imagine yourself drawing in positive energy and strength, and with each exhale, release any negative thoughts or emotions that may be weighing you down.

Step-by-step guide for practicing Anchoring Breathing:

1. Find a quiet and comfortable space: Begin by finding a quiet, comfortable space where you can sit or lie down. Ensure that you won't be disturbed during your practice.

2. Take a few deep breaths: Take a few deep breaths, inhaling deeply through your nose and exhaling slowly through your mouth. This will help you relax and prepare for the practice.

3. Choose an image or physical anchor: Choose an image or physical anchor to focus on during the practice. This could be a meaningful phrase, a mental image, or a physical object such as a crystal or piece of jewelry.

4. Visualize or focus on your anchor: Close your eyes and visualize your chosen image or focus on the physical sensation of your anchor. With each inhale, imagine yourself drawing in positive energy and strength, and with each exhale, release any negative thoughts or emotions that may be weighing you down.

5. Repeat: Continue to breathe deeply and focus on your anchor for 5-10 minutes, or longer if desired. As you finish the practice, take a few deep breaths and open your eyes slowly, bringing your awareness back to your surroundings.

Remember to take your time and adjust the practice to your personal preferences and needs. With regular practice, Anchoring Breathing can be a powerful tool for reducing stress, increasing focus, and promoting emotional wellbeing.

Case studies or personal anecdotes: While there are no specific case studies on Anchoring Breathing, many individuals have reported positive results from practicing this technique, including increased feelings of relaxation, greater mental clarity, and improved mood and emotional regulation.

Scientific research and studies: There is limited scientific research on Anchoring Breathing specifically, but studies have shown that deep breathing and visualization techniques can have a positive impact on stress and anxiety levels, as well as cognitive performance and overall well-being.

Cultural and spiritual origins: Anchoring Breathing does not have any specific cultural or spiritual origins, but many spiritual and mindfulness practices incorporate deep breathing and visualization techniques to promote relaxation and focus.

Practical tips and exercises for daily practice: To incorporate Anchoring Breathing into your daily routine, set aside a few minutes each day to practice deep breathing and visualization. Choose a comfortable, quiet space and a time when you can fully focus on the practice. Experiment with different visualizations or physical anchors until you find one that resonates with you.

Precautions and contraindications: Anchoring Breathing is generally safe for most individuals, but it is important to listen to your body and stop the practice if you experience any discomfort or pain. Individuals with respiratory conditions should consult with a healthcare professional before practicing deep breathing techniques.

Further resources and recommendations: For more information on Anchoring Breathing and other breathing techniques, consider seeking out a qualified mindfulness or meditation teacher, or consult with a healthcare professional for personalized guidance.

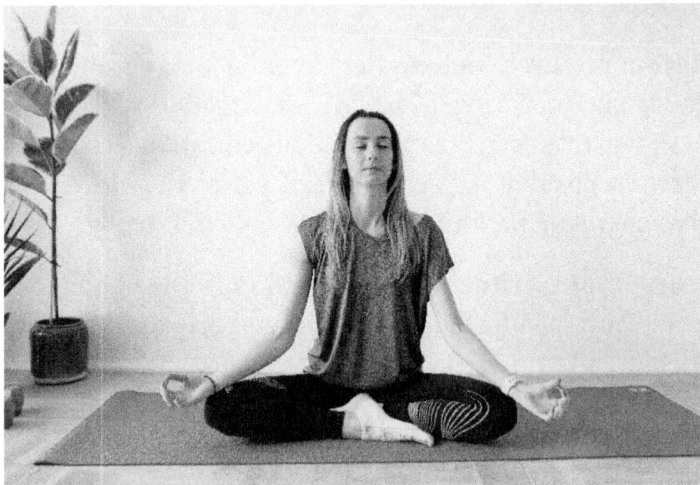

Anchoring Breathing

By Melody Wallack

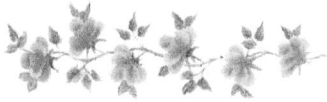

Inhale, exhale, find your ground,

Feel your feet on solid earth,

Breathe in peace, breathe out doubt,

Your anchor in the stormy surf.

***

Let your breath be your guide,

As you navigate life's rough seas,

With each inhale, let peace reside,

With each exhale, release what no longer serves.

***

Anchor your breath, anchor your soul,

As you face each new day,

Let the rhythm of your breath console,

And carry you through in every way.

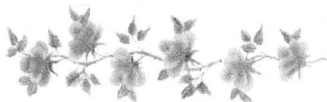

6.Box Breathing (Square Breathing or 4x4 Breathing - Sama Vritti)

Box breathing, also known as Sama Vritti, is a simple yet powerful technique used to calm the mind and reduce stress. It involves inhaling for a certain count, holding the breath for the same count, exhaling for the same count, and holding the breath again for the same count. The even count of inhalation, retention, exhalation, and retention gives it the name "box breathing."

History and Origins: Box breathing is a technique that has been used in many different cultures and traditions for thousands of years. It is commonly associated with yoga and meditation practices, where it is used to help calm the mind and increase focus. The technique has also been used by military personnel and athletes to manage stress and improve performance.

Specific Benefits: Box breathing has been shown to have a number of physical and mental benefits. It can help to reduce stress and anxiety, lower blood pressure, improve digestion, enhance focus and concentration, and promote feelings of calm and relaxation. It is also thought to stimulate the parasympathetic nervous system, which is responsible for promoting relaxation and rest.

Variations and Techniques: The basic technique of box breathing involves inhaling for a count of four, holding the breath for a count of four, exhaling for a count of four, and holding the breath again for a count of four. However, there are many variations that can be used to adapt the technique to an individual's needs or preferences. For example, the counts can be lengthened or shortened, the breath can be held for a longer or shorter period of time, and the technique can be combined with other practices, such as visualization or mantra repetition.

Step-by-step guide on how to practice Box Breathing:

1. Find a quiet, comfortable space where you can sit or lie down. Sit with your back straight and your feet planted firmly on the ground, or lie down on your back with your arms at your sides.

2. Close your eyes and take a few deep breaths, inhaling deeply through your nose and exhaling slowly through your mouth. Try to relax your body and clear your mind of any distractions.

3. Visualize a box in your mind's eye. Imagine that the box has four sides, each representing a different stage of the breathing exercise.

4. Inhale deeply for a count of four: Begin by inhaling slowly through your nose, counting to four in your head. Focus on filling your lungs with air and expanding your belly.

5. Hold the breath for a count of four: Once you have taken a full inhale, hold your breath for a count of four.

6. Exhale for a count of four: Slowly exhale through your mouth, counting to four in your head. Focus on releasing all the air from your lungs.

7. Hold the breath for a count of four: Once you have fully exhaled, hold your breath for a count of four before beginning the next inhale.

8. Repeat the cycle: Repeat this cycle of inhaling, holding, exhaling, and holding for several minutes. Start with practicing for 1-2 minutes and gradually increase the duration over time.

You can also experiment with different counts that work for you. **For example**, you might try *inhaling for a count of six, holding for a count of two, exhaling for a count of six, and holding for a count of two.*

To enhance the benefits of box breathing, you can combine it with other practices, such as visualization or mantra repetition. **For example**, *you might visualize a peaceful scene or repeat a positive affirmation during each cycle of breath.*

With regular practice, box breathing can help reduce stress and anxiety, improve focus and concentration, and promote relaxation and a sense of calm.

Case Studies or Personal Anecdotes: Many individuals have reported experiencing significant benefits from practicing box breathing. For example, some individuals have reported that it has helped them to manage symptoms of anxiety and depression, while others have found it useful for improving their athletic performance or managing stress in high-pressure situations.

Scientific Research and Studies: There is limited scientific research on the benefits of box breathing specifically, but studies have shown that similar breathing techniques, such as slow and deep breathing, can help to reduce stress and anxiety, lower blood pressure, and improve overall well-being.

Cultural and Spiritual Origins: Box breathing has its roots in various spiritual and cultural traditions, including yoga, martial arts, and mindfulness practices. It is often used as a tool for developing greater self-awareness and promoting spiritual growth.

Practical Tips and Exercises for Daily Practice: Box breathing can be practiced anywhere, anytime, and by anyone. To practice, find a comfortable seated position and begin by taking a few deep breaths. Then, inhale for a count of four, hold for a count of four, exhale for a count of four, and hold again for a count of four. Repeat this cycle for several minutes, gradually lengthening the counts if desired. It can be helpful to focus on the sensation of the breath as it moves in and out of the body, and to visualize the breath moving in a square or box shape.

Precautions and Contraindications: Box breathing is generally safe for most individuals, but it is important to listen to your body and not push yourself beyond your limits. If you experience any discomfort or dizziness, slow down or stop the practice altogether. Individuals with certain medical conditions, such as asthma or heart disease, should consult with their healthcare provider before trying this technique.

Further Resources and Recommendations: For more information on box breathing and other breathing techniques, there are many resources available, including books, online courses, and workshops. It can also be helpful to work with a qualified teacher or healthcare provider to develop a safe and effective breathing practice.

7.Alternate nostril breathing (Nadi Shodhana)

Alternate nostril breathing, also known as Nadi Shodhana or Anulom Vilom Pranayama, is a breathing technique that has been used in traditional Indian medicine for centuries. It involves breathing through one nostril at a time while closing the other nostril with the fingers.

History and origins: Nadi Shodhana is a Sanskrit term for *"channel cleansing."* This technique is believed to balance the flow of prana, or life force energy, through the body's energy channels. Nadi Shodhana has been used for thousands of years in the practice of yoga, Ayurveda, and other traditional Indian healing systems.

Specific benefits: Alternate nostril breathing is believed to calm the mind, reduce stress and anxiety, and promote overall well-being. It may also help to balance the two hemispheres of the brain and improve cognitive function. Some practitioners believe that Nadi Shodhana can help to purify the energy channels in the body and balance the flow of prana.

Variations and techniques: To perform alternate nostril breathing, sit comfortably with your spine straight and your eyes closed. Use your right hand to block your right nostril with your thumb and inhale deeply through your left nostril. Then, use your ring finger or little finger to block your left nostril and exhale through your right nostril. Inhale again through your right nostril, then block your right nostril and exhale through your left nostril. This is one cycle of alternate nostril breathing. Repeat for several minutes, gradually increasing the duration of each inhale and exhale.

Step-by-step instruction for alternate nostril breathing:

1. Find a comfortable seated position: Sit comfortably with your spine straight and your eyes closed.

2. Use your right hand to block your right nostril: Curl your right index and middle fingers toward your palm and use your thumb to block your right nostril.

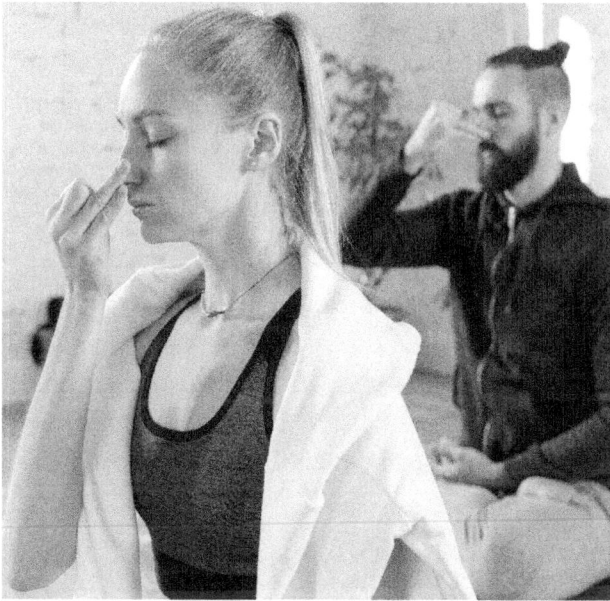

3. Inhale deeply through your left nostril: Gently and slowly inhale through your left nostril for a count of 4-6 seconds.

4. Block your left nostril and exhale through your right nostril: Release the thumb from your right nostril and use your ring finger or little finger to block your left nostril. Exhale slowly and completely through your right nostril for a count of 4-6 seconds.

5. Inhale through your right nostril: Keeping your left nostril blocked, inhale slowly and deeply through your right nostril for a count of 4-6 seconds.

6. Block your right nostril and exhale through your left nostril: Release your left nostril and use your thumb to block your right nostril. Exhale slowly and completely through your left nostril for a count of 4-6 seconds.

7. Repeat: This completes one cycle of alternate nostril breathing. Repeat steps 3-6 for several minutes, gradually increasing the duration of each inhale and exhale.

    Note: Always start with the left nostril inhale and end with the left nostril exhale.

Case studies or personal anecdotes: Many people report feeling more relaxed and centered after practicing alternate nostril breathing. Some also find that it helps to clear the mind and improve mental focus. However, more scientific research is needed to fully understand the benefits of this technique.

Scientific research and studies: Studies have shown that alternate nostril breathing can help to reduce stress and improve heart rate variability, a measure of the balance between the sympathetic and parasympathetic nervous systems. It may also help to improve lung function and reduce symptoms of asthma.

Cultural and spiritual origins: Alternate nostril breathing has been practiced for thousands of years in traditional Indian medicine and yoga. It is believed to balance the flow of prana, or life force energy, through the body's energy channels.

Practical tips and exercises for daily practice: To incorporate alternate nostril breathing into your daily routine, try practicing for 5-10 minutes each day, gradually increasing the duration over time. It can be helpful to set aside a dedicated time and place for your practice, such as in the morning or before bed. If you are new to this technique, it may be helpful to work with a teacher or guide to ensure proper technique and avoid potential complications.

Precautions and contraindications: People with certain medical conditions, such as chronic obstructive pulmonary disease (COPD), should consult with a healthcare provider before practicing alternate nostril breathing. It may also be contraindicated for individuals with certain nasal or sinus conditions.

Further resources and recommendations: There are many resources available for learning and practicing alternate nostril breathing, including books, videos, and online courses. It may be helpful to work with a qualified teacher or guide to ensure proper technique and avoid potential complications.

8.Buteyko Breathing

History and Origins: Buteyko breathing was developed by Ukrainian physiologist Konstantin Buteyko in the 1950s. Buteyko noticed that people who breathed shallowly and with less volume seemed to have better health outcomes than those who breathed more deeply and frequently. He hypothesized that hyperventilation caused a reduction in carbon dioxide in the blood, leading to a host of health problems. Buteyko developed a set of breathing exercises designed to reduce the volume and frequency of breathing in order to increase the amount of carbon dioxide in the blood.

Specific Benefits: Buteyko breathing has been used to treat a range of health conditions, including asthma, chronic obstructive pulmonary disease (COPD), anxiety, and sleep apnea. The technique is thought to improve the efficiency of breathing and increase oxygen delivery to the tissues. Additionally, Buteyko breathing may help to reduce symptoms of stress and anxiety by promoting relaxation and reducing hyperventilation.

Variations and Techniques: Buteyko breathing involves a series of breathing exercises that aim to reduce the volume and frequency of breathing. The technique involves slow, shallow breathing through the nose with relaxed exhalation. The exercises are typically performed sitting or standing, and may involve breath holds or pauses. Buteyko breathing also emphasizes the importance of nasal breathing, as opposed to mouth breathing.

Step-by-step instruction for Buteyko breathing technique:

1. Sit or stand in a comfortable position with your back straight.

2. Close your mouth and breathe in slowly and gently through your nose, focusing on filling your lower lungs with air.

3. Exhale slowly and gently through your nose, allowing your lungs to empty completely.

4. Pause briefly after each exhale before taking your next inhale.

5. Repeat steps 2-4 for several minutes, gradually increasing the duration of each inhale and exhale.

6. You can also incorporate breath holds or pauses in your practice by exhaling completely and holding your breath for a few seconds before taking your next inhale.

Remember to keep your breathing slow, shallow, and relaxed throughout the practice. Emphasize nasal breathing, keeping your mouth closed as much as possible. With regular practice, Buteyko breathing can help reduce the volume and frequency of your breathing, leading to improved overall health and wellbeing.

Case Studies or Personal Anecdotes: Many people have reported success in using Buteyko breathing to manage asthma symptoms and improve lung function. One case study published in the Journal of Asthma and Allergy found that practicing Buteyko breathing for four weeks led to improvements in asthma symptoms, medication use, and lung function in a group of asthmatic patients. However, more research is needed to confirm these findings.

Scientific Research and Studies: While there is some evidence to suggest that Buteyko breathing may be effective in improving lung function and reducing symptoms of asthma and other respiratory conditions, more research is needed to confirm these findings. A 2019 systematic review of Buteyko breathing for asthma found that while the technique may be effective in reducing symptoms and improving lung function, more high-quality studies are needed to confirm these results.

Cultural and Spiritual Origins: Buteyko breathing does not have any specific cultural or spiritual origins, as it was developed by a medical researcher in the 1950s.

Practical Tips and Exercises for Daily Practice: Buteyko breathing exercises can be practiced throughout the day, and may be particularly helpful during times of stress or anxiety. One simple exercise involves taking a deep breath in through the nose, followed by a slow, relaxed exhalation through the nose. The exhale should be longer than the inhale, and should be accompanied by a feeling of relaxation and release.

Precautions and Contraindications: Buteyko breathing is generally considered safe for most people, but it is important to consult with a healthcare provider before starting any new breathing or exercise program. Additionally, people with certain health conditions, such as low blood pressure or heart disease, may need to modify the technique or avoid certain exercises.

Further Resources and Recommendations: For more information on Buteyko breathing, resources and recommendations can be found on the Buteyko Clinic International website and in the book "Close Your Mouth: Buteyko Clinic Handbook for Perfect Health."

9.Pursed Lip Breathing

History and Origins: Pursed lip breathing is a simple breathing technique that has been used for centuries to help people with respiratory conditions such as chronic obstructive pulmonary disease (COPD), asthma, and emphysema. It is thought to have originated in ancient India and was later adopted by Western medicine.

Specific Benefits: Pursed lip breathing can help to slow down breathing, reduce shortness of breath, and increase oxygen levels in the body. It can also help to reduce the amount of air trapped in the lungs and make breathing more efficient. This technique has been found to be especially helpful for people with COPD, as it can improve their exercise tolerance and quality of life.

Variations and Techniques: To practice pursed lip breathing, first, inhale deeply through your nose for 2-3 seconds. Then, purse your lips as if you are about to whistle or blow out a candle, and exhale slowly through your pursed lips for 4-6 seconds. The exhalation should be twice as long as the inhalation. This technique can be repeated for several breaths or as long as necessary to feel comfortable.

Step-by-step instruction for pursed lip breathing:

1. Sit comfortably with your back straight and your shoulders relaxed.

2. Inhale deeply through your nose for 2-3 seconds.

3. Purse your lips as if you are about to whistle or blow out a candle.

4. Exhale slowly and steadily through your pursed lips for 4-6 seconds.

5. Focus on the feeling of the air passing through your lips and on the sensation of the exhale.

6. Repeat the process for several breaths or as long as necessary to feel comfortable.

Case Studies or Personal Anecdotes: A study published in the Journal of Cardiopulmonary Rehabilitation and Prevention found that pursed lip breathing can significantly improve shortness of breath and exercise tolerance in people with COPD. Another study published in the Journal of Physical Therapy Science found that pursed lip breathing can improve lung function and reduce respiratory rate in people with asthma.

Scientific Research and Studies: Research has shown that pursed lip breathing can improve lung function, reduce shortness of breath, and improve exercise tolerance in people with COPD and other respiratory conditions. It has also been found to be effective in reducing anxiety and promoting relaxation in healthy individuals.

Cultural and Spiritual Origins: Pursed lip breathing is not traditionally associated with any specific culture or spiritual practice. However, it is often used in yoga and meditation practices as a way to improve breathing and increase relaxation.

Practical Tips and Exercises for Daily Practice: Pursed lip breathing can be practiced anywhere, anytime, and is an excellent technique for managing shortness of breath during daily activities or exercise. To get the most benefit from pursed lip breathing, try practicing it for 5-10 minutes a day, several times a day.

Precautions and Contraindications: Pursed lip breathing is generally safe and can be practiced by people of all ages and fitness levels. However, if you experience any discomfort or pain while practicing this technique, stop and seek medical advice.

Further Resources and Recommendations: For more information on pursed lip breathing and its benefits, consult with your healthcare provider or a certified respiratory therapist. There are also many online resources available, including instructional videos and breathing exercises.

10. Ocean breathing or Victorious Breath (Ujjayi)

Ocean breathing, also known as Ujjayi, is a yogic breathing technique that involves breathing deeply and slowly through the nose while constricting the back of the throat to create a gentle hissing or ocean-like sound. This technique is commonly used in yoga practices, but can also be used outside of yoga for relaxation and stress relief.

History and origins: Ujjayi breathing has been practiced in yoga for thousands of years and is believed to have originated in ancient India. The word "ujjayi" comes from the Sanskrit language and means "victorious" or "triumphant," representing the benefits and power of the technique.

Specific benefits: Ujjayi breathing has been found to have numerous benefits, including:

- Relieving stress and anxiety

- Improving concentration and mental focus

- Enhancing physical performance and endurance

- Stimulating the parasympathetic nervous system and promoting relaxation

- Increasing lung capacity and oxygenation

- Regulating blood pressure and heart rate

Variations and techniques: Ujjayi breathing involves inhaling and exhaling deeply through the nose, while constricting the back of the throat to create a hissing or ocean-like sound. This sound can be amplified or decreased depending on the level of constriction in the throat. There are variations in the technique, such as adjusting the length and speed of the breath or incorporating it into different yoga poses.

Step-by-step guide for Ujjayi breathing:

1. Find a comfortable seated or lying position: Ujjayi breathing can be practiced in any comfortable position, such as seated cross-legged or lying down.

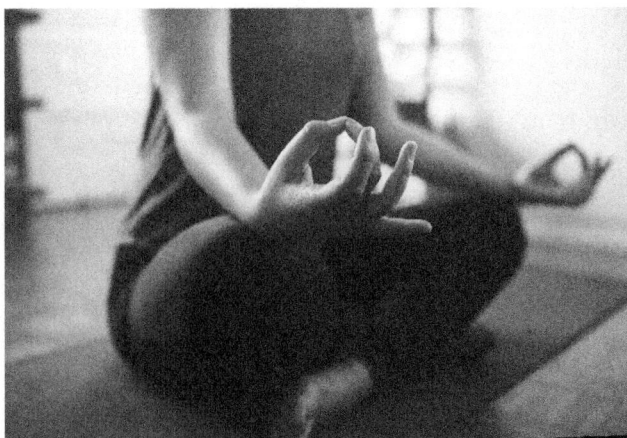

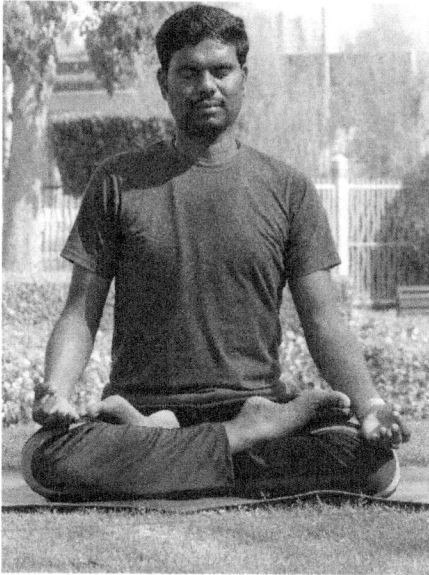

2. Inhale deeply through your nose: Take a slow, deep breath in through your nose, filling your lungs completely.

3. Constrict the back of your throat: As you exhale, constrict the muscles at the back of your throat, as if you are fogging up a mirror. This will create a hissing or ocean-like sound in the back of your throat.

4. Focus on the sound: Pay attention to the sound of the breath, using it as a focal point for your concentration.

5. Inhale and exhale deeply: Continue breathing deeply through your nose, constricting the back of your throat on the exhale to create the sound.

6. Vary the length and speed: Experiment with different lengths and speeds of the breath to find what works best for you. You can also try incorporating Ujjayi breathing

into different yoga poses, such as sun salutations or warrior poses.

7. Practice regularly: Aim to practice Ujjayi breathing for a few minutes each day, gradually increasing the duration of your practice over time. With regular practice, you may notice improved concentration, reduced stress and anxiety, and increased relaxation.

Case studies or personal anecdotes: Many individuals have reported experiencing a sense of calm and relaxation after practicing Ujjayi breathing, as well as improved concentration and focus. Some athletes have also reported using the technique to increase their endurance and improve their performance.

Scientific research and studies: There is limited scientific research specifically on Ujjayi breathing, but studies on deep breathing and yogic breathing techniques have found similar benefits, such as reducing stress and anxiety, improving lung function, and enhancing athletic performance.

Cultural and spiritual origins: Ujjayi breathing is deeply rooted in the cultural and spiritual traditions of yoga, which originated in ancient India. The technique is often used as a way to connect with the breath and calm the mind during yoga practice.

Practical tips and exercises for daily practice: To practice Ujjayi breathing, find a comfortable seated position and inhale deeply through the nose while constricting the back of the throat to create a gentle hissing or ocean-like sound. Hold the breath briefly, and then exhale slowly through the nose while continuing to make the same sound. Start with a few rounds of Ujjayi breathing and gradually increase the duration and intensity of the breath as comfortable.

Precautions and contraindications: Ujjayi breathing is generally considered safe for most individuals, but it may not be suitable for those with certain respiratory conditions, such as asthma or chronic obstructive pulmonary disease (COPD). It is important to consult with a healthcare provider before starting a new breathing practice.

Further resources and recommendations: For more information on Ujjayi breathing and other breathing techniques, there are many resources available, such as yoga classes, books, and online tutorials. Some recommended resources include "Light on Yoga" by B.K.S. Iyengar, "The Breathing Book" by Donna Farhi, and online yoga classes and tutorials from Yoga Journal and Yoga International.

11. Dirga Pranayama Breathing

History and Origins: Dirga Pranayama is a yogic breathing technique with roots in ancient Indian texts. The word "Dirga" means "long," and "Pranayama" refers to the practice of breath control. This technique is believed to have been developed thousands of years ago as a way to balance the body and mind and prepare for deeper meditation.

Specific Benefits: Dirga Pranayama is a calming and centering breathing technique that helps to reduce stress and anxiety. This technique can improve lung function, increase oxygenation, and improve overall respiratory health. It is also believed to stimulate the parasympathetic nervous system, promoting relaxation and reducing symptoms of depression.

Variations and Techniques: Dirga Pranayama involves breathing in three parts - the belly, the lower ribs, and the upper chest.

Step-by-step instructions for practicing Dirga Pranayama:

1. Find a comfortable seated position with your back straight and your eyes closed.

2. Place one hand on your belly and the other on your chest.

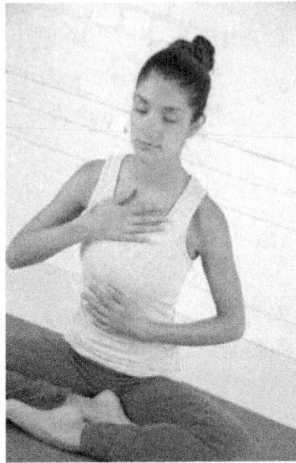

3. Take a deep breath in through your nose, allowing your belly to expand as you inhale.

4. Continue to inhale, expanding your lower ribs and then your upper chest.

5. Hold the breath for a few seconds.

6. Exhale slowly, first releasing the air from your chest, then your ribs, and finally your belly.

7. Repeat the cycle, focusing on breathing into each part of your body - the belly, lower ribs, and upper chest - as you inhale, and releasing the air slowly as you exhale.

Case Studies or Personal Anecdotes: Many people who practice Dirga Pranayama report feeling more calm and centered after just a few minutes of practice. Some individuals have reported significant improvements in their lung function and respiratory health after incorporating Dirga Pranayama into their daily routine.

Scientific Research and Studies: Research has shown that practicing Dirga Pranayama can have a positive impact on the respiratory system, including increased lung function and oxygenation. Additionally, this technique has been found to reduce stress and anxiety levels and improve symptoms of depression.

Cultural and Spiritual Origins: Dirga Pranayama is a widely practiced technique in the yogic tradition, originating in ancient India. It is often used as a preparation for meditation and other spiritual practices, as it helps to calm the mind and body.

Practical Tips and Exercises for Daily Practice: To incorporate Dirga Pranayama into your daily routine, try practicing for a few minutes each day in a quiet, comfortable space. Focus on breathing deeply and slowly, expanding your belly, lower ribs, and upper chest with each inhalation. Try to hold the breath for a few seconds before exhaling slowly and fully.

Precautions and Contraindications: While Dirga Pranayama is generally considered safe for most people, those with respiratory conditions such as asthma should speak with a healthcare professional before beginning this practice. It is also important to practice Dirga Pranayama in a safe and comfortable environment and to avoid overexerting the breath.

Further Resources and Recommendations: For more information on Dirga Pranayama and other yogic breathing techniques, consider seeking guidance from a qualified yoga teacher or respiratory therapist. There are also many resources available online and in books on the topic of breathwork and yogic practices.

12. Skull shining breath (Kapalabhati)

History and origins: Kapalabhati is a pranayama technique that originates from traditional Indian yogic practices. The word Kapalabhati is derived from two Sanskrit words, "Kapala" which means skull and "bhati" which means shining. The technique involves rapid, forceful exhalations and passive inhalations, often accompanied by abdominal contractions.

Specific benefits: Kapalabhati is believed to have numerous physical and mental health benefits. It is said to help improve digestion, stimulate the metabolism, and enhance lung function. It may also help improve mental clarity, reduce stress and anxiety, and increase overall energy levels.

Variations and techniques: There are several variations of Kapalabhati, but the basic technique involves sitting in a comfortable, upright position with the eyes closed.

Here are the step-by-step instructions for Kapalabhati:

1. Find a comfortable seated position with your spine straight and your eyes closed.

2. Take a few deep breaths in and out through your nose to relax and center yourself.

3. Inhale deeply through your nose and exhale forcefully and rapidly through your nose while simultaneously contracting your abdominal muscles.

4. The inhale should be passive and relaxed, with the belly naturally expanding as you inhale.

5. Repeat this cycle of forceful exhales and passive inhales for several rounds, gradually increasing the speed and intensity of the exhales.

6. Start with 10-20 rounds and gradually work your way up to 100 or more rounds, depending on your experience and comfort level.

7. After completing the rounds, take a few deep breaths in and out through your nose to return to a normal breathing pattern.

8. You can practice Kapalabhati for a few minutes each day, gradually increasing the duration and intensity of the practice over time.

Case studies or personal anecdotes: One case study published in the International Journal of Yoga found that regular practice of Kapalabhati helped improve respiratory function in patients with asthma. Another study published in the Journal of Ayurveda and Integrative Medicine found that Kapalabhati was effective in reducing stress and anxiety levels in healthy adults.

Scientific research and studies: There is limited scientific research on the effectiveness of Kapalabhati, but some studies suggest that it may have benefits for respiratory function, stress reduction, and cognitive function. More research is needed to fully understand the potential benefits and risks of this technique.

Cultural and spiritual origins: Kapalabhati is deeply rooted in traditional Indian yogic practices and is often used in conjunction with other pranayama techniques and asanas in yoga practice. It is believed to help purify the body and mind, and increase the flow of prana or life force energy.

Practical tips and exercises for daily practice: Kapalabhati should be practiced on an empty stomach, preferably in the morning. It is important to start with slow, controlled exhales and gradually increase the speed and intensity over time. It is also important to maintain a relaxed and focused state of mind during the practice.

Precautions and contraindications: Kapalabhati should be avoided by individuals with high blood pressure, heart disease, epilepsy, and other medical conditions. It may also be contraindicated during pregnancy and menstruation. It is important to consult with a healthcare professional before starting this or any other breathing technique.

Further resources and recommendations: For further guidance and instruction on Kapalabhati and other pranayama techniques, consider working with a qualified yoga teacher or pranayama instructor. There are also many resources available online and in books on the practice of pranayama and yogic breathing techniques.

13. Breath of fire (Kapalabhati)

History and origins: Breath of fire, or Kapalabhati, is a traditional breathing technique that originated in India. The term "Kapalabhati" is derived from the Sanskrit words "kapala" meaning "skull" and "bhati" meaning "shine" or "illuminate." It is believed to have been practiced by yogis and sages in ancient India as a way to purify the mind and body.

Specific benefits: Breath of fire is said to provide a wide range of benefits, including:

- Increasing oxygen intake and improving respiratory function

- Stimulating digestion and detoxification

- Boosting energy levels and enhancing mental clarity

- Balancing the nervous system and reducing stress and anxiety

- Strengthening the abdominal muscles and improving core stability

Variations and techniques: Breath of fire involves rapid, forceful exhales through the nose, while the inhales are passive and automatic. To perform the technique, sit in a comfortable position with the spine straight and the hands on the knees or in the lap. Inhale deeply and then begin to forcefully exhale through the nose in short bursts, pumping the belly in towards the spine with each exhale. The inhales should happen naturally, without any effort or force. The pace should be fast and rhythmic, with each round consisting of 20-30 exhales.

Step-by-step guide for performing Breath of Fire:

1. Sit in a comfortable position with your spine straight and your hands resting on your knees or lap.

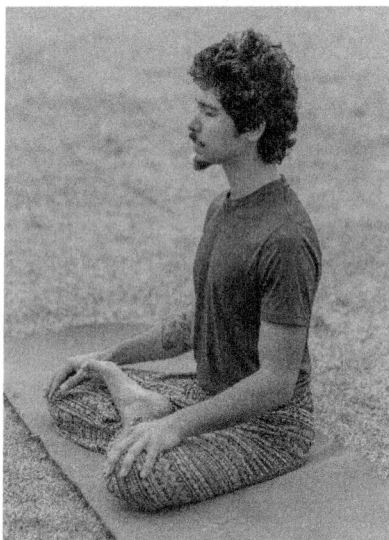

2. Take a deep inhale through your nose.

3. Begin forcefully exhaling through your nose in short, rhythmic bursts, pumping your belly in towards your spine with each exhale.

4. Allow the inhales to happen naturally, without any effort or force.

5. Maintain a fast and rhythmic pace, with each round consisting of 20-30 exhales.

6. Practice for 1-3 minutes, gradually increasing the duration over time.

7. After completing the practice, take a few deep breaths and allow your body to relax.

Note: Breath of Fire is an advanced breathing technique and should be avoided by individuals with certain medical conditions, such as high blood pressure or glaucoma. Consult with a healthcare professional before practicing this technique.

Case studies or personal anecdotes: Many individuals have reported experiencing benefits from practicing breath of fire. For example, some people report feeling more energized and focused after practicing the technique, while others have reported improvements in their digestion and overall health.

Scientific research and studies: Research on the specific effects of breath of fire is limited, but studies have found that pranayama (breathing) practices in general can have positive effects on respiratory function, blood pressure, and stress reduction.

Cultural and spiritual origins: Breath of fire is a common practice in yoga and is often included in Kundalini yoga kriyas (sequences). It is believed to help awaken the inner fire, or "agni," and purify the mind and body.

Practical tips and exercises for daily practice: Breath of fire can be practiced on its own or as part of a longer yoga or meditation practice. To begin, start with a few rounds of 20-30 exhales, gradually building up to longer rounds and more repetitions. It is important to keep the inhales passive and relaxed, allowing the body to naturally take in air. If you experience dizziness or lightheadedness, take a break and return to normal breathing.

Precautions and contraindications: Breath of fire is generally safe for most people to practice, but it is not recommended for individuals with high blood pressure, heart conditions, or respiratory problems. Women who are pregnant should also avoid practicing breath of fire.

Further resources and recommendations: For more information on breath of fire and how to practice it safely, consult with a certified yoga instructor or pranayama teacher. There are also numerous books and online resources available on the topic of pranayama and breathwork.

14. Cooling Breathing (Sitali Breath)

Sitali Pranayama is a cooling breathing technique that has been used in traditional yoga practices for centuries. Here is a detailed overview of its history, variations, benefits, and more:

History and Origins: Sitali Pranayama is a Sanskrit term that translates to "cooling breath." It is believed to have originated in ancient India and was traditionally used to cool the body and calm the mind during hot summer months. The practice involves inhaling air through the mouth, which is then passed over the tongue and throat to create a cooling effect.

Specific Benefits: Sitali Pranayama is believed to have a variety of physical and mental benefits. Some of these include:

- Cooling the body and reducing inflammation
- Lowering blood pressure and heart rate
- Reducing stress and anxiety
- Improving digestion
- Boosting the immune system
- Enhancing mental clarity and focus

Variations and Techniques: To practice Sitali Pranayama, sit in a comfortable cross-legged position with your hands on your knees or in your lap. Open your mouth slightly and roll your tongue into a tube-like shape, then inhale slowly and deeply through your mouth. As you inhale, focus on the cooling sensation created by the air passing over your tongue and throat. After inhaling fully, close your mouth and exhale slowly through your nose. Repeat for several rounds.

Step-by-step instruction for Sitali Pranayama:

1. Sit comfortably in a cross-legged position with your hands on your knees or in your lap.

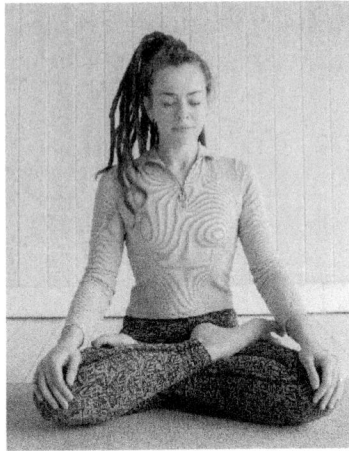

2. Open your mouth slightly and roll your tongue into a tube-like shape. If you are unable to roll your tongue, you can purse your lips instead.

3. Inhale slowly and deeply through your mouth, focusing on the cooling sensation created by the air passing over your tongue and throat.

4. After inhaling fully, close your mouth and exhale slowly through your nose.

5. Repeat for several rounds, inhaling through your mouth and exhaling through your nose each time.

6. You can start with five rounds and gradually increase the number of rounds as you become more comfortable with the practice.

If you are unable to roll your tongue into a tube-like shape, you can also practice Sitali Pranayama by pursing your lips and inhaling through the mouth as if sipping through a straw.

Case Studies or Personal Anecdotes: While there is limited scientific research on the specific benefits of Sitali Pranayama, many practitioners have reported positive effects on their physical and mental health. Some have even reported using the practice to lower fever and reduce the symptoms of heatstroke.

Scientific Research and Studies: Limited scientific research has been conducted on the effects of Sitali Pranayama. However, a small study published in the International Journal of Yoga found that the practice may have a positive effect on blood pressure and heart rate in individuals with hypertension.

Cultural and Spiritual Origins: Sitali Pranayama has been traditionally used in the practice of yoga and is considered a cooling and calming practice. It is often used in combination with other breathing techniques and physical postures to balance the body and mind.

Practical Tips and Exercises for Daily Practice: To incorporate Sitali Pranayama into your daily routine, try practicing the technique for several rounds before or after your yoga practice, or any time you need to cool down or calm your mind. As with any breathing practice, start with a few rounds and gradually increase the duration and frequency over time.

Precautions and Contraindications: Sitali Pranayama is generally safe for most people to practice. However, if you have any respiratory issues or difficulty breathing through the nose, consult with a healthcare provider before attempting this practice. It is also important to practice Sitali

Pranayama in a cool, well-ventilated space and avoid practicing in extreme heat or humidity.

Further Resources and Recommendations: For more information on Sitali Pranayama and other breathing techniques, consider exploring resources on traditional yoga practices or consulting with a certified yoga teacher or healthcare provider. There are also numerous online resources and mobile apps that offer guided breathing exercises and mindfulness practices.

15.Humming bee breath (Bhramari) Breathing

History and origins: Humming bee breath, also known as Bhramari Pranayama, is a breathing technique that has been practiced in yoga for thousands of years. Its origins can be traced back to ancient India, where it was believed to have numerous health benefits for both the mind and body.

Specific benefits: Humming bee breath is known to have a calming effect on the mind and body, helping to reduce stress and anxiety. It can also improve concentration, increase mental clarity, and improve overall mood.

Variations and techniques: To practice humming bee breath, begin by sitting comfortably with your eyes closed. Take a deep breath in, and as you exhale, make a humming sound with your lips closed. You can also place your fingers on your ears and gently press to create a resonating effect. Repeat this several times, taking deep breaths in between each round.

Step-by-step instructions for humming bee breath:

1. Get into a comfortable seated position with your back straight and your eyes closed.

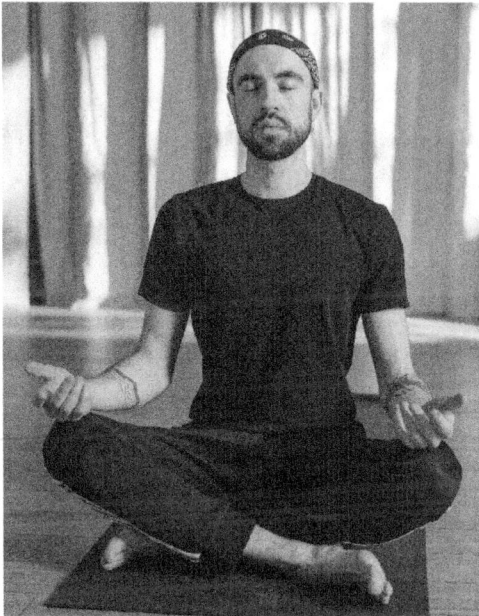

2. Take a deep breath in through your nose, filling your lungs with air.

3. As you exhale, close your lips and make a humming sound.

4. Keep your lips closed and continue to hum as you exhale completely.

5. Repeat this process for several rounds, taking deep breaths in between each round.

6. If desired, you can also place your fingers on your ears and gently press to create a resonating effect.

Note: It is important to take breaks as needed and stop the practice if you feel any discomfort or dizziness. Try to do 20 minutes a day for eight weeks.

Case studies or personal anecdotes: Many individuals who practice humming bee breath report feeling more relaxed and centered, with a greater sense of inner peace and tranquility. Some people also report that it helps to relieve symptoms of anxiety, depression, and insomnia.

Scientific research and studies: While there is limited scientific research specifically on humming bee breath, studies on other forms of pranayama (yogic breathing) have shown promising results. One study found that practicing pranayama techniques, including humming bee breath, for just **20 minutes a day for eight weeks** led to a significant reduction in symptoms of anxiety and depression.

Cultural and spiritual origins: In traditional yoga practice, humming bee breath is often used in conjunction with meditation and other yogic practices to promote spiritual growth and development. It is believed to help awaken the energy centers in the body, or chakras, leading to a greater sense of inner peace and connection to the divine.

Practical tips and exercises for daily practice: To incorporate humming bee breath into your daily routine, try practicing it first thing in the morning or before bed. You can also use it as a tool to help calm your mind and body during stressful situations throughout the day.

Precautions and contraindications: While humming bee breath is generally considered safe for most individuals, those with certain medical conditions, such as ear infections or tinnitus, should avoid the technique. As with any new exercise or breathing practice, it is always best to consult with a healthcare provider before beginning.

Further resources and recommendations: For those interested in learning more about humming bee breath and other pranayama techniques, there are numerous resources available online, including instructional videos and guided meditations. Consider attending a yoga or meditation class to learn directly from a teacher experienced in these practices.

Humming bee breath (Bhramari)

By Melody Wallack

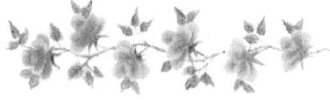

As the buzz of the bee fills the air,
I close my eyes and begin to prepare.
Inhale, exhale, and let out a hum,
Feeling the vibrations, a sense of calm.
***
With each breath, I release the stress,
The worries, the fears, the endless mess.
I focus on the sound, the gentle drone,
Feeling the peace that I have known.
***
The bee becomes a part of me,
A tool to set my mind free.
With each hum, I find my way,
To a place of stillness, come what may.
***
Oh humming bee, you show the way,
To a world of peace, day by day.
I breathe with you, I hum with you,
And find the calm that I once knew.

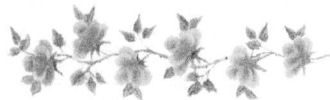

16. Coherent Breathing

History and Origins: Coherent breathing has roots in the ancient yogic practice of pranayama, which emphasizes the control and manipulation of the breath to improve physical and mental health. Coherent breathing specifically was developed in the 1970s by Dr. Richard Brown and Dr. Patricia Gerbarg as a technique to help regulate the body's stress response and promote relaxation.

Specific benefits: Research has shown that coherent breathing can improve heart rate variability, a measure of the flexibility and resilience of the cardiovascular system. It has also been found to reduce symptoms of anxiety, depression, and post-traumatic stress disorder (PTSD). Additionally, coherent breathing may help regulate the body's stress response and improve sleep quality.

Variations and techniques: Coherent breathing involves inhaling and exhaling at a rate of six breaths per minute, or five seconds inhale and five seconds exhale. This can be achieved by counting silently to five for both inhalation and exhalation, or by using a visual cue such as a metronome. The technique can be practiced in a seated or lying down position.

Step-by-step instructions for coherent breathing:

1. Find a comfortable seated or lying down position. You can sit in a chair with your feet flat on the floor, or lie down on your back with your arms at your sides.

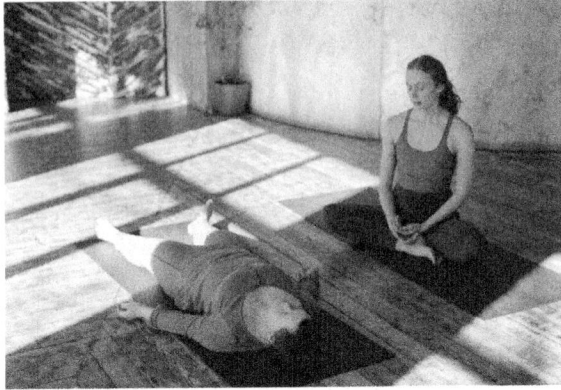

2. Close your eyes and begin to breathe in and out through your nose. Allow your breath to be natural and easy.

3. Begin to inhale for a count of five seconds. You can count silently to yourself or use a visual cue like a metronome to keep track of the time.

4. Hold your breath for a count of one or two seconds.

5. Exhale for a count of five seconds. Again, you can count silently or use a visual cue to keep track of the time.

6. Hold your breath for one or two seconds.

7. Repeat this pattern of inhaling for five seconds, holding for one or two seconds, exhaling for five seconds, and holding for one or two seconds. Try to maintain a steady, rhythmic pace.

8. Practice for 5-10 minutes, gradually increasing the duration of your practice as you become more comfortable with the technique.

Note: It's important to maintain a relaxed and gentle pace with coherent breathing. If you find that you're feeling lightheaded or uncomfortable, slow down the pace or take a break from the practice.

Case studies or personal anecdotes: One study found that practicing coherent breathing for 20 minutes a day for four weeks led to significant improvements in symptoms of depression and anxiety in college students. Another study found that coherent breathing reduced symptoms of PTSD in veterans.

Scientific research and studies: A study published in the Journal of Alternative and Complementary Medicine found that coherent breathing reduced symptoms of depression and anxiety in college students. Another study published in the Journal of Traumatic Stress found that coherent breathing reduced symptoms of PTSD in veterans.

Cultural and spiritual origins: Coherent breathing has roots in the ancient practice of pranayama in yoga, which emphasizes the control and manipulation of the breath to improve physical and mental health.

Practical tips and exercises for daily practice: To practice coherent breathing, inhale for a count of five, then exhale for a count of five. Repeat for 10-20 minutes daily.

Precautions and contraindications: Coherent breathing is generally considered safe for most people, but those with certain health conditions, such as cardiovascular disease, should consult with a healthcare professional before practicing.

Further resources and recommendations: Brown, R. P., Gerbarg, P. L., & Muench, F. (2013). Breathing practices for treatment of psychiatric and stress-related medical conditions. Psychiatric Clinics, 36(1), 121-140. Gerritsen, R. J., & Band, G. P. (2018). Breath of life: The respiratory vagal stimulation model of contemplative activity. Frontiers in Human Neuroscience, 12, 397. Gerritsen, R. J., & Band, G. P. (2018). Vagus nerve function in relation to cognitive and affective processes. Journal of Psychophysiology, 32(1), 1-14.

17.Lion's Breathing (Simhasana)

Lion's breath, also known as Simhasana, is a yogic breathing technique that is said to relieve tension and stress in the face, neck, and chest. It involves a forceful exhalation with an open mouth and a distinctive roar-like sound.

History and origins: Lion's breath has its origins in the ancient practice of yoga. It is believed to have been developed as a way to release tension and pent-up emotions and to stimulate the throat chakra, which is associated with self-expression and communication.

Specific benefits: Lion's breath is said to have numerous benefits, including:

- Relieving tension and stress in the face, neck, and chest

- Stimulating the throat chakra and promoting self-expression

- Improving focus and concentration

- Reducing anxiety and depression

- Boosting the immune system by increasing oxygen flow to the body

Variations and techniques: To practice lion's breath, sit in a comfortable cross-legged position with your hands resting on your knees or thighs. Take a deep breath in through your nose, then exhale forcefully through your mouth while sticking out your tongue and making a "haaa" sound. Imagine you are roaring like a lion as you exhale. Repeat this for several rounds, taking deep breaths in between.

Step-by-step instructions for practicing lion's breath:

1. Sit in a comfortable cross-legged position with your hands resting on your knees or thighs.

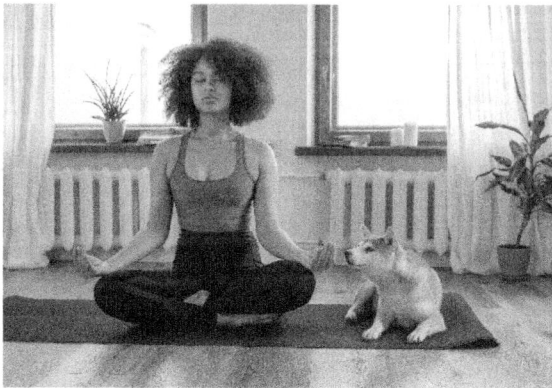

2. Take a deep breath in through your nose.

3. Exhale forcefully through your mouth while sticking out your tongue as far as it can go.

4. As you exhale, make a "haaa" sound as if you are roaring like a lion.

5. Imagine you are letting go of any tension, stress, or negative emotions as you exhale.

6. Repeat for several rounds, taking deep breaths in between.

7. You can also try variations of lion's breath, such as holding the tongue out and rolling the eyes up towards the third eye while exhaling, or taking a deep breath in and then exhaling while sticking out the tongue and opening the eyes wide.

Note: Some variations of lion's breath include holding the tongue out and rolling the eyes up towards the third eye while exhaling, or taking a deep breath in and then exhaling while sticking out the tongue and opening the eyes wide.

Case studies or personal anecdotes: While there is limited research on the specific benefits of lion's breath, many practitioners have reported experiencing reduced stress and increased energy after practicing this technique regularly.

Scientific research and studies: There is limited scientific research on lion's breath specifically, but studies have shown that similar breathing techniques, such as diaphragmatic breathing, can have a positive impact on stress, anxiety, and depression.

Cultural and spiritual origins: Lion's breath has its roots in yoga and is often practiced in conjunction with other yoga poses and meditation. It is said to help release pent-up emotions and connect the practitioner with their inner strength and courage.

Practical tips and exercises for daily practice: Lion's breath can be practiced anytime, anywhere, and is especially useful during times of stress or anxiety. Try incorporating this technique into your daily yoga or meditation practice, or practice it for a few rounds whenever you need a quick energy boost.

Precautions and contraindications: Lion's breath is generally considered safe for most people, but it may not be suitable for those with respiratory issues or high blood pressure. As with any new exercise or breathing technique, it is best to consult with a healthcare provider before beginning.

Further resources and recommendations: To learn more about lion's breath and other yogic breathing techniques, consider taking a yoga class or seeking out resources online or at your local library. The book "Light on Pranayama" by B.K.S. Iyengar is a comprehensive guide to the practice of pranayama, including lion's breath and other techniques.

18. Tummo Breathing (Inner Fire)

Tummo breathing, also known as Inner Fire breathing, is a breathing technique that originates from the Tibetan Buddhist tradition. The practice is based on the belief that through breathing and meditation, one can awaken the inner fire or heat within the body.

History and Origins: Tummo breathing has been practiced by Tibetan Buddhist monks for centuries. It is believed to have originated from the teachings of Indian yogis and was later incorporated into Tibetan Buddhist practices.

Specific Benefits: Tummo breathing is said to have numerous benefits, including increased energy, improved focus and concentration, reduced stress and anxiety, and improved physical health. Some practitioners also believe that the practice can help with the treatment of certain medical conditions.

Variations and Techniques: Tummo breathing involves various techniques, including deep breathing exercises, visualization, and meditation. One common method involves sitting cross-legged and focusing on the breath, while visualizing flames in the lower belly. The practitioner then focuses on raising the heat and energy up through the body.

Step-by-step instruction for Tummo breathing:

1. Find a comfortable seated position: Sit cross-legged on a cushion or mat with your back straight and your hands resting on your knees or in your lap.

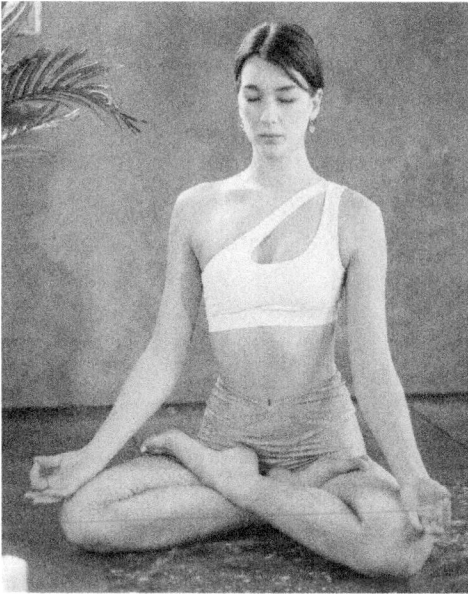

2. Take a few deep breaths: Inhale deeply through your nose and exhale slowly through your mouth, allowing yourself to relax and become centered.

3. Visualize flames in the lower belly: Imagine a flame burning in your lower belly, just below the navel. Focus on the warmth and energy of the flame.

4. Inhale deeply and contract the pelvic floor: As you inhale, contract your pelvic floor muscles and visualize the flame growing brighter and hotter.

5. Hold the breath: Hold the breath for a few seconds while visualizing the flame spreading up through your body.

6. Exhale slowly and relax: Release the pelvic floor contraction and exhale slowly through your nose, visualizing the flame receding back down to the lower belly.

7. Repeat the process: Continue practicing Tummo breathing, focusing on the visualization and the flow of energy through your body.

   Note: It is important to approach Tummo breathing with caution and under the guidance of a qualified teacher, as it involves advanced techniques that can be potentially dangerous if practiced improperly.

Case Studies or Personal Anecdotes: There are many personal anecdotes of the benefits of Tummo breathing, including increased energy levels, improved physical health, and improved mental clarity and focus.

Scientific Research and Studies: Limited scientific research has been conducted on Tummo breathing. However, one study conducted on Tibetan monks showed that they were able to increase their body temperature through the practice of Tummo meditation.

Cultural and Spiritual Origins: Tummo breathing is deeply rooted in Tibetan Buddhist culture and is considered to be a spiritual practice.

Practical Tips and Exercises for Daily Practice: To incorporate Tummo breathing into daily practice, individuals can start with basic breathing exercises and gradually work up to more advanced techniques. It is important to work with a qualified teacher to ensure proper technique and safety.

Precautions and Contraindications: Tummo breathing is not recommended for individuals with certain medical conditions, such as high blood pressure or heart disease. It is important to consult with a healthcare provider before starting any new breathing or meditation practices.

Further Resources and Recommendations: Resources for learning and practicing Tummo breathing include books, online tutorials, and qualified teachers in the Tibetan Buddhist tradition. It is important to approach this practice with respect and to work with a qualified teacher to ensure safe and effective practice.

19. Holotropic Breathwork

History and Origins: Holotropic Breathwork is a modern method of breathwork that was developed by Stanislav Grof, a Czech psychiatrist, in the 1970s. Grof initially created Holotropic Breathwork as a way to explore the potential of non-ordinary states of consciousness in therapy, drawing on his research into LSD-assisted psychotherapy. Over time, Holotropic Breathwork has evolved into a therapeutic technique in its own right, used to access deep states of consciousness and promote personal growth and healing.

Specific Benefits: Holotropic Breathwork is believed to promote personal growth and healing by accessing and integrating suppressed emotions and memories, releasing physical tension and trauma, and connecting with spiritual and transpersonal dimensions of consciousness.

Variations and Techniques: Holotropic Breathwork typically involves breathing rapidly and deeply for an extended period, often accompanied by music or other sensory stimuli. Participants are encouraged to let go of control and allow the breath to guide them into altered states of consciousness. The experience is usually facilitated by trained practitioners who provide support and guidance throughout the process.

Step-by-step instructions for Holotropic Breathwork:

1. Find a quiet, comfortable space: Holotropic Breathwork is usually done in a group setting, so find a quiet, comfortable space where you won't be disturbed.

2. Get into a comfortable position: Lie down on your back or sit upright with your back straight. Use pillows or blankets to support your body and make yourself as comfortable as possible.

3. Begin breathing rapidly and deeply: Start breathing deeply and rapidly, focusing on filling your lungs with air and exhaling fully. Use your diaphragm to breathe deeply and rhythmically, without pausing between inhalations and exhalations.

4. Allow the breath to guide you: As you continue breathing, let go of control and allow the breath to guide you. You may begin to feel sensations in your body or experience visualizations or emotions.

5. Allow the experience to unfold: Stay with the breath and allow the experience to unfold naturally. Trust the process and allow whatever needs to come up to come up.

6. End the session: When you feel ready to end the session, slow your breathing down and take a few deep, slow breaths. Gently open your eyes and take a few moments to ground yourself before getting up.

Note: It is highly recommended to do Holotropic Breathwork with a trained practitioner who can provide support and guidance throughout the process. It is also important to ensure that you are in good physical and mental health before trying this technique.

Case Studies or Personal Anecdotes: Many people who have tried Holotropic Breathwork report transformative experiences, including profound spiritual insights, emotional release, and physical healing. However, as with any powerful therapeutic technique, it is important to approach Holotropic Breathwork with caution and work with trained practitioners who can guide you through the process safely.

Scientific Research and Studies: There is limited scientific research on the efficacy of Holotropic Breathwork, but anecdotal evidence suggests that it can be a powerful tool for personal growth and healing when used in a safe and supportive environment.

Cultural and Spiritual Origins: Holotropic Breathwork draws on various spiritual and therapeutic traditions, including shamanism, transpersonal psychology, and Eastern meditation practices. It is not affiliated with any specific cultural or religious tradition.

Practical Tips and Exercises for Daily Practice: Holotropic Breathwork is typically practiced in a group setting, facilitated by trained practitioners. It is not recommended to attempt Holotropic Breathwork on your own without proper training and guidance.

Precautions and Contraindications: Holotropic Breathwork can be a powerful and transformative experience, but it is not suitable for everyone. People with certain medical or psychiatric conditions, such as high blood pressure or bipolar disorder, may be advised to avoid Holotropic Breathwork. It is important to work with trained practitioners who can assess your individual needs and provide appropriate guidance and support.

Further Resources and Recommendations: For more information on Holotropic Breathwork, you can visit the website of the Grof Foundation (https://www.stanislavgrof.com/). The foundation offers training programs for Holotropic Breathwork facilitators, as well as resources for those interested in exploring this therapeutic technique.

20. Equal breathing or 2-to-1 breathing

2-to-1 breathing, also known as Sama Vritti, is a simple yet effective breathing technique that involves inhaling for a count of two and exhaling for a count of four. This technique is commonly used in yoga, meditation, and mindfulness practices to promote relaxation and reduce stress.

History and Origins: The origins of 2-to-1 breathing can be traced back to ancient yogic texts. It is a fundamental breathing technique taught in yoga classes and is commonly used in pranayama (breathing) practices to balance the body and mind. The technique has been used for thousands of years to promote physical and mental health.

Specific Benefits: The 2-to-1 breathing technique has been shown to have numerous benefits for both physical and mental health. Some of the specific benefits include:

- Reducing stress and anxiety: The slow and rhythmic breathing pattern helps to activate the parasympathetic nervous system, which promotes relaxation and reduces stress and anxiety.

- Lowering blood pressure: Regular practice of 2-to-1 breathing has been shown to lower blood pressure and improve cardiovascular health.

- Improving lung function: The controlled breathing pattern of 2-to-1 breathing can help to increase lung capacity and improve respiratory function.

- Enhancing focus and concentration: The breathing technique helps to calm the mind and increase mental clarity, making it a useful tool for enhancing focus and concentration.

Variations and Techniques: The basic technique of 2-to-1 breathing involves inhaling for two counts and exhaling for four counts. This can be practiced in a seated or lying-down position, with the eyes closed or open. One variation is to gradually increase the length of the inhale and exhale, for example, inhaling for three counts and exhaling for six counts.

Step-by-step for practicing 2-to-1 breathing:

1. Find a comfortable seated or lying-down position: You can sit on a cushion or chair with your back straight or lie down on your back.

2. Close your eyes or keep them open if you prefer.

3. Inhale for two counts: Take a deep breath in through your nose, counting to two.

4. Exhale for four counts: Slowly exhale through your nose, counting to four. Focus on releasing all the air from your lungs.

5. Repeat: Continue inhaling for two counts and exhaling for four counts. You can start with a few rounds and gradually increase the number of rounds as you feel comfortable.

6. Increase the length of the inhale and exhale: Once you are comfortable with the basic technique, you can gradually increase the length of your inhale and exhale. For example, you can inhale for three counts and exhale for six counts.

7. Practice daily: Incorporate 2-to-1 breathing into your daily routine. You can do it first thing in the morning, during a break at work, or before bed to help you relax.

Note: Remember to breathe deeply and stay focused on your breath as you practice.

Another variation is to add a brief pause at the top of the inhale and bottom of the exhale. This is known as breath retention or Kumbhaka, and it can help to increase lung capacity and improve oxygenation.

Case Studies or Personal Anecdotes: There are many personal anecdotes and case studies that attest to the effectiveness of 2-to-1 breathing for reducing stress and promoting relaxation. Many individuals report feeling calmer and more centered after just a few minutes of practicing this technique.

Scientific Research and Studies: Several scientific studies have investigated the effects of 2-to-1 breathing on physical and mental health. One study published in the International Journal of Yoga Therapy found that regular practice of 2-to-1 breathing can significantly reduce anxiety and depression symptoms in patients with cardiovascular disease. Another study published in the Journal of Clinical and Diagnostic Research found that practicing 2-to-1 breathing can improve lung function in healthy individuals.

Cultural and Spiritual Origins: 2-to-1 breathing has its roots in ancient yogic traditions and is often taught in yoga classes as a basic breathing technique. It is also commonly used in mindfulness and meditation practices.

Practical Tips and Exercises for Daily Practice: To practice 2-to-1 breathing, find a comfortable seated or lying-down position and close your eyes. Inhale for a count of two, then exhale for a count of four. Repeat for several minutes, gradually increasing the length of the inhale and exhale as you become more comfortable. You can also add a brief pause at the top of the inhale and bottom of the exhale.

Precautions and Contraindications: 2-to-1 breathing is generally safe for most individuals, but it is important to listen to your body and not push yourself beyond your limits. If you experience dizziness or discomfort while practicing this technique, slow down or stop and return to normal breathing.

Further Resources and Recommendations: For more information on 2-to-1 breathing and other breathing techniques, there are a variety of resources available, including books, workshops, and online courses. Here are some recommendations:

1. "The Science of Breath" by Swami Rama, Rudolph Ballentine, and Alan Hymes - This book provides a comprehensive overview of various breathing techniques and their benefits, including 2-to-1 breathing.

2. "Breathe: The Simple, Revolutionary 14-Day Program to Improve Your Mental and Physical Health" by Belisa Vranich - This book offers practical tips and exercises for incorporating breathing techniques into daily life, including 2-to-1 breathing.

3. Online courses and workshops - Many yoga studios and wellness centers offer workshops and courses on breathing techniques, including 2-to-1 breathing. Check with your local studio or center for upcoming offerings.

4. Breathing apps - There are several apps available that provide guided breathing exercises, including 2-to-1 breathing. Some popular options include Prana Breath, Breathe+, and Breathing Zone.

Remember to consult with a healthcare professional before beginning any new breathing practice, especially if you have any pre-existing health conditions. With regular practice and proper guidance, 2-to-1 breathing can be a powerful tool for improving overall health and well-being.

2-to-1 Breathing (Sama Vritti)

By Melody Wallack

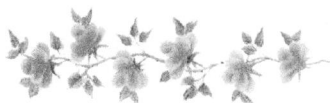

Inhale for two, exhale for four

The rhythm of life, forevermore

Breath flowing in and out with ease

Bringing calmness, a sense of peace

With each inhale, feel the power

Of life and energy, in this hour

And with each exhale, let go

Of all that weighs us down below

In this practice of Sama Vritti

We find a state of inner serenity

A stillness in the midst of life's storms

A place where we can be reborn.

21. Wim Hof Method

History and origins: The Wim Hof Method is a breathing technique developed by Wim Hof, also known as "The Iceman," who has set multiple world records for withstanding extreme cold. Hof developed this method based on his personal experiences with cold exposure and meditation.

Specific benefits: The Wim Hof Method has been reported to improve a range of health outcomes, including reduced inflammation, improved immune function, increased energy levels, and reduced stress and anxiety. It has also been associated with improvements in conditions such as asthma, arthritis, and autoimmune disorders.

Variations and techniques: The Wim Hof Method involves a combination of breathing exercises, cold exposure, and meditation. The breathing technique involves taking deep breaths in and out in a rhythmic manner, followed by holding the breath for a period of time. This cycle is repeated multiple times, and can be done for several rounds. The cold exposure component involves gradually exposing the body to cold temperatures, such as taking cold showers or submerging in ice baths. Meditation is also a key component of the method, and can be used to focus the mind and promote relaxation.

Step-by-step instruction is for the Wim Hof Method.

1. Find a comfortable place to sit or lie down: Find a comfortable position either sitting or lying down. Ensure that you are in a relaxed and comfortable state.

2. Take 30-40 deep breaths: Take 30-40 deep breaths in a rhythmic manner. Inhale deeply through your nose, then

exhale through your mouth without forcing the breath out.

3. Hold the breath: After completing the deep breaths, exhale and hold your breath for as long as you comfortably can.

4. Take another deep breath and hold: Inhale deeply through your nose, then exhale and hold your breath again for as long as you comfortably can.

5. Repeat: Repeat the cycle for several rounds, gradually increasing the duration of the breath holds.

6. Cold exposure: Gradually expose the body to cold temperatures, such as taking cold showers or submerging in ice baths. Start with short periods of cold exposure and gradually increase the duration over time.

7. Meditation: Practice meditation to focus the mind and promote relaxation. This can be done in combination with the breathing and cold exposure components of the method.

Case studies or personal anecdotes: There are numerous personal anecdotes from individuals who have experienced benefits from practicing the Wim Hof Method, including increased resilience to cold temperatures and improved mental and physical health.

Scientific research and studies: Although more research is needed, there is some scientific evidence to support the benefits of the Wim Hof Method. For example, a 2014 study found that practicing the method resulted in decreased inflammation and increased immune response in participants. Another study published in 2018 reported improvements in mood, energy levels, and sleep quality among individuals who practiced the method regularly.

Cultural and spiritual origins: The Wim Hof Method does not have specific cultural or spiritual origins, but it does draw on principles from Eastern practices such as yoga and meditation.

Practical tips and exercises for daily practice: To practice the Wim Hof Method, it is recommended to start with a guided course or instructor to learn the proper techniques and safety precautions. The method can be adapted to individual preferences and needs, but a basic routine may involve several rounds of the breathing exercise, followed by a cold shower or exposure to cold temperatures, and then meditation.

Precautions and contraindications: The Wim Hof Method involves exposure to cold temperatures, which may not be suitable for individuals with certain health conditions, such as cardiovascular disease or Raynaud's syndrome. It is important to consult with a healthcare provider before starting this practice.

Further resources and recommendations: There are many resources available for individuals interested in learning more about the Wim Hof Method, including books, online courses, and workshops. It is recommended to seek out qualified instructors and to approach this practice with caution and mindfulness.

In conclusion, the 21 breathing techniques detailed in this chapter offer a variety of options for individuals seeking to improve their physical, mental, and emotional well-being through the power of the breath. While each technique has its own specific benefits and variations, it's important to remember that not every technique will work for every person. Therefore, we recommend starting with the five techniques mentioned above: *diaphragmatic breathing, Zen breathing, relaxing breathing, stimulating breathing, and anchoring breathing*. As you continue to practice and explore these techniques, you may discover which ones resonate most with you and incorporate them into your daily routine. Remember, consistent practice is key to reaping the full benefits of these techniques.

Chapter 4

Breathing Techniques for Relaxation and Stress Relief

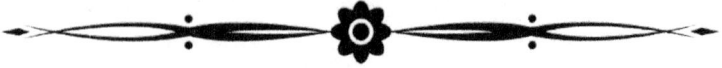

1. **Diaphragmatic Breathing (Belly Breathing)**

   a) Description: Diaphragmatic breathing involves engaging the diaphragm while allowing the belly to expand and contract with each breath. This technique promotes deep, slow breathing, which helps activate the parasympathetic nervous system and promotes relaxation.

   b) Instructions: Sit or lie down in a comfortable position. Place one hand on your chest and the other on your belly. Inhale deeply through your nose, allowing your belly to expand while keeping your chest relatively still. Exhale slowly through your mouth or nose, feeling your belly contract. Continue this pattern for several minutes, focusing on the rise and fall of your belly.

2. **4-7-8 Breathing (Relaxing Breath)**

   a) Description: The 4-7-8 breathing technique is a simple practice that involves inhaling for a count of 4, holding the breath for a count of 7, and exhaling for a count of 8. This technique helps to slow down the breath and activate the relaxation response.

b) b. Instructions: Sit or lie down in a comfortable position with your back straight. Close your eyes and begin by exhaling fully through your mouth. Inhale quietly through your nose for a count of 4. Hold your breath for a count of 7. Exhale through your mouth for a count of 8, making a gentle whooshing sound. Repeat this cycle for a total of four breaths.

3. **Box Breathing (Square Breathing)**

   a) Description: Box breathing, also known as square breathing, is a technique that involves inhaling, holding the breath, exhaling, and holding the breath again, all for equal counts. This practice helps to regulate the breath and promote relaxation.

   b) Instructions: Sit or lie down in a comfortable position with your back straight. Close your eyes and take a few deep, cleansing breaths. Begin by inhaling slowly and deeply through your nose for a count of 4. Hold your breath for a count of 4. Exhale slowly through your mouth or nose for a count of 4. Hold your breath again for a count of 4. Repeat this cycle for several minutes.

4. **Progressive Muscle Relaxation (PMR) and Breathing**

   a) Description: Progressive muscle relaxation (PMR) is a technique that involves tensing and relaxing various muscle groups while focusing on the breath. This practice helps to release physical tension and promote overall relaxation.

b) Instructions: Sit or lie down in a comfortable position. Close your eyes and take a few deep breaths. Begin by tensing a specific muscle group, such as your feet or hands, as you inhale. Hold the tension for a few seconds, then release and relax the muscles as you exhale. Move through each muscle group, tensing and relaxing as you breathe in and out.

5. **Guided Imagery and Breathing**

   a) Description: Guided imagery is a technique that involves visualizing peaceful, calming scenes or images while focusing on the breath. This practice can help reduce stress, promote relaxation, and improve mood.

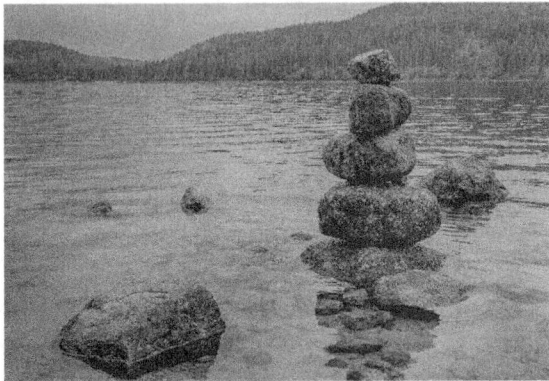

   b) b. Instructions: Sit or lie down in a comfortable position with your eyes closed. Take a few deep, cleansing breaths. Begin to visualize a peaceful scene, such as a beach, forest, or mountain landscape. Focus on the details of the scene and allow yourself to become immersed in the experience. Breathe deeply and slowly as you continue to visualize the calming imagery.

These five techniques are just a few examples of the many breathing practices that can help promote relaxation and stress relief. It's essential to explore different techniques to find the ones that resonate with you and best suit your needs. As you continue to practice these techniques regularly, you will likely notice improvements in your overall stress levels and emotional well-being.

In the subsequent sections, we will discuss other categories of breathing techniques that focus on different aspects of well-being, such as increasing energy and focus, promoting balance and mindfulness, and addressing specific health conditions.

As you incorporate these breathing practices into your daily routine, remember that consistency is key. Regular practice can help train your body and mind to respond more effectively to stress, improving your resilience and overall quality of life.

When practicing these techniques, it's important to remember that each person's experience may vary. Some individuals may find certain techniques more effective or enjoyable than others. Therefore, it is essential to remain open to trying different approaches and discovering what works best for you in terms of relaxation and stress relief.

In the following sections of the book, we will dive deeper into the various breathing techniques designed for specific purposes and needs. As you explore these techniques, you will likely find that your understanding of your breath and its impact on your well-being continues to grow, empowering you to take control of your health and emotional state through the power of conscious breathing.

Chapter 5

Breathing Techniques for Energy and Focus

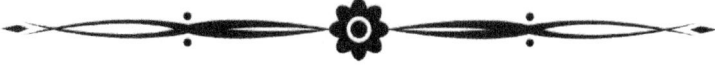

1. **Stimulating Breath (Bellows Breath)**

   a) Description: The stimulating breath, also known as bellows breath or Bhastrika Pranayama in yoga, is a technique that involves rapid, forceful inhales and exhales through the nose. This practice helps to energize the body, increase mental alertness, and improve focus.

   b) Instructions: Sit in a comfortable position with your back straight. Close your eyes and take a few deep, cleansing breaths. Begin to inhale and exhale rapidly through your nose, using your diaphragm to create short, powerful breaths. Keep the inhales and exhales equal in duration, aiming for about three breaths per second. Practice for up to 15 seconds initially, gradually increasing the duration as you become more comfortable with the technique.

2. **Alternate Nostril Breathing (Nadi Shodhana Pranayama)**

   a) Description: Alternate nostril breathing, also known as Nadi Shodhana Pranayama, is a yoga technique that involves inhaling through one nostril, holding the breath, and exhaling through the other nostril. This practice helps to balance the left and right hemispheres of the brain, promote mental clarity, and increase focus.

b) Instructions: Sit in a comfortable position with your back straight. Close your eyes and take a few deep, cleansing breaths. Using your right hand, place your thumb on your right nostril and your ring finger on your left nostril. Close your right nostril with your thumb and inhale slowly through your left nostril. Close your left nostril with your ring finger, and hold your breath for a moment. Release your thumb from your right nostril and exhale slowly. Inhale through your right nostril, close it with your thumb, hold your breath, and then exhale through your left nostril. This completes one cycle. Repeat for several minutes.

3. **Breath of Fire (Kapalabhati Pranayama)**
   a) Description: Breath of Fire, also known as Kapalabhati Pranayama, is a yoga technique that involves rapid, forceful exhales through the nose while engaging the abdominal muscles. This practice helps to energize the body, stimulate the brain, and improve focus.

   b) Instructions: Sit in a comfortable position with your back straight. Close your eyes and take a few deep, cleansing breaths. Begin to exhale rapidly through your nose, using your abdominal muscles to push the air out. Allow the inhales to occur passively as your abdomen relaxes. Focus on the forceful exhales and maintain a steady rhythm, aiming for about one exhale per second. Practice for up to one minute, gradually increasing the duration as you become more comfortable with the technique.

4. Ujjayi Breathing (Victorious Breath or Ocean Breath)

a) Description: Ujjayi breathing, also known as victorious breath or ocean breath, is a yoga technique that involves inhaling and exhaling through the nose while slightly constricting the back of the throat. This practice creates a soothing sound, similar to ocean waves, and helps to calm the mind, improve concentration, and increase energy.

b) Instructions: Sit in a comfortable position with your back straight. Close your eyes and take a few deep, cleansing breaths. Begin to inhale through your nose, slightly constricting the back of your throat to create a gentle hissing sound. Exhale through your nose, maintaining the constriction in your throat and creating the same hissing sound. Continue to breathe in this way, focusing on the soothing sound and sensation of the breath as it moves through your throat. Practice for several minutes, gradually increasing the duration as you become more comfortable with the technique.

5. Sitali Pranayama (Cooling Breath)

a) Description: Sitali Pranayama, also known as the cooling breath, is a yoga technique that involves inhaling through a curled tongue and exhaling through the nose. This practice helps to cool the body, calm the mind, and increase mental clarity and focus.

b) Instructions: Sit in a comfortable position with your back straight. Close your eyes and take a few deep, cleansing breaths. Curl your tongue into a tube-like shape, extending it slightly out of your mouth. Inhale slowly through your curled tongue, drawing cool air into your mouth and down into your lungs. Close your mouth, hold your breath for a moment, and then exhale slowly through your nose. Repeat this process for several minutes.

6. **Humming Bee Breath (Bhramari Pranayama)**

   a) Description: The humming bee breath, also known as Bhramari Pranayama, is a yoga technique that involves inhaling through the nose and exhaling while creating a humming sound. This practice helps to calm the mind, reduce stress, and improve concentration and focus.

   b) Instructions: Sit in a comfortable position with your back straight. Close your eyes and take a few deep, cleansing breaths. Place your index fingers on the cartilage between your cheeks and ears. Inhale deeply through your nose, and as you exhale, create a humming sound by gently vibrating the back of your throat. Keep your mouth closed and feel the vibrations in your head and face. Continue to breathe in this way, focusing on the soothing sound and sensation of the humming vibrations. Practice for several minutes, gradually increasing the duration as you become more comfortable with the technique.

As you explore these techniques for energy and focus, remember that each person's experience may vary. Some individuals may find certain techniques more effective or enjoyable than others. Therefore, it is essential to remain open to trying different approaches and discovering what works best for you in terms of energizing your body and sharpening your mind.

In the following sections of the book, we will delve into breathing techniques for balance and mindfulness, as well as those designed to address specific health conditions. With consistent practice and a willingness to explore a variety of techniques, you will continue to deepen your understanding of the transformative power of the breath and its impact on your overall well-being.

Chapter 6

Breathing Techniques for Balance and Mindfulness

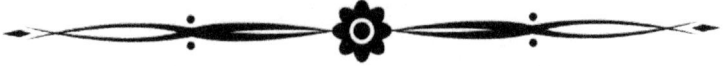

1. **Diaphragmatic Breathing (Abdominal Breathing)**

   a) Description: Diaphragmatic breathing, also known as abdominal breathing, is a technique that involves inhaling deeply and slowly through the nose, allowing the diaphragm to expand and the abdomen to rise. This practice helps to promote relaxation, reduce stress, and cultivate mindfulness.

   b) Instructions: Sit or lie down in a comfortable position with your back straight. Place one hand on your chest and the other on your abdomen. Close your eyes and take a few deep, cleansing breaths. Begin to inhale slowly and deeply through your nose, focusing on expanding your abdomen as you breathe. Exhale slowly through your nose, allowing your abdomen to contract. Continue to breathe in this way, maintaining a slow and steady rhythm and keeping your focus on the movement of your abdomen. Practice for several minutes, gradually increasing the duration as you become more comfortable with the technique.

2. **Mindful Breathing (Observing the Breath)**

   a) Description: Mindful breathing is a simple meditation technique that involves observing the breath without judgment or trying to control it. This practice helps to cultivate mindfulness, improve focus, and develop a greater awareness of the present moment.

b) Instructions: Sit in a comfortable position with your back straight. Close your eyes and take a few deep, cleansing breaths. Begin to observe your natural breathing rhythm without trying to change or control it. Notice the sensation of the breath as it enters and exits your nostrils, the rise and fall of your chest and abdomen, and any other sensations associated with your breath. If your mind begins to wander, gently bring your focus back to your breath. Practice for several minutes, gradually increasing the duration as you become more comfortable with the technique.

3. **Four-Seven-Eight Breathing (Relaxing Breath)**

a) Description: The 4-7-8 breathing technique, also known as the relaxing breath, is a practice that involves inhaling for a count of four, holding the breath for a count of seven, and exhaling for a count of eight. This technique helps to promote relaxation, reduce stress, and improve emotional balance.

b) Instructions: Sit in a comfortable position with your back straight. Close your eyes and take a few deep, cleansing breaths. Begin to inhale slowly through your nose for a count of four. Hold your breath for a count of seven. Exhale slowly through your mouth for a count of eight, making a gentle whooshing sound as you release the breath. Repeat this cycle for a total of four breaths, gradually increasing the number of cycles as you become more comfortable with the technique.

4. **Box Breathing (Square Breathing)**

a) Description: Box breathing, also known as square breathing, is a technique that involves inhaling, holding the breath, exhaling, and holding the breath again, all for equal counts. This practice helps to promote relaxation, improve focus, and cultivate mindfulness.

b) Instructions: Sit in a comfortable position with your back straight. Close your eyes and take a few deep, cleansing breaths. Begin to inhale slowly through your nose for a count of four. Hold your breath for a count of four. Exhale slowly through your mouth for a count of four. Hold your breath again for a count of four. Repeat this cycle for several minutes, gradually increasing the duration as you become more comfortable with the technique.

5. **Three-Part Breath (Dirga Pranayama)**

a) Description: The three-part breath, also known as Dirga Pranayama, is a yoga technique that involves inhaling deeply into the abdomen, ribcage, , and upper chest in a sequential manner. This practice helps to promote relaxation, improve lung capacity, and cultivate mindfulness.

b) Instructions: Sit or lie down in a comfortable position with your back straight. Close your eyes and take a few deep, cleansing breaths. Begin to inhale slowly through your nose, focusing on filling your abdomen with air. Once your abdomen is full, continue to inhale as you expand your ribcage. Finally, complete your inhalation by filling your upper chest with air. Exhale slowly and completely through your nose, releasing the air from your upper chest, ribcage, and abdomen in reverse order. Continue to breathe in this three-part manner for several minutes, gradually increasing the duration as you become more comfortable with the technique.

6. **Alternate Nostril Breathing (Nadi Shodhana Pranayama)**

a) Description: Alternate nostril breathing, also known as Nadi Shodhana Pranayama, is a yoga technique that involves inhaling and exhaling through one nostril at a time while alternately blocking the other nostril. This practice helps to balance the left and right hemispheres of the brain, reduce stress, and promote mental clarity and focus.

b) Instructions: Sit in a comfortable position with your back straight. Close your eyes and take a few deep, cleansing breaths. Using your right thumb, gently close your right nostril. Inhale slowly through your left nostril. At the top of your inhalation, use your right ring finger to close your left nostril and release your thumb from your right nostril. Exhale slowly through your right nostril. Inhale through your right nostril, then close it with your thumb and release your ring finger from your left nostril. Exhale through your left nostril. This completes one cycle of alternate nostril breathing. Continue to practice for several minutes, gradually increasing the duration as you become more comfortable with the technique.

These six techniques for balance and mindfulness can be practiced individually or combined to create a comprehensive breathwork practice that supports mental, emotional, and physical well-being. By consistently incorporating these techniques into your daily routine, you will develop a greater sense of balance, awareness, and mindfulness in your life.

In the next section, we will explore breathing techniques specifically designed to address various health conditions. Through targeted breathwork, you can harness the power of your breath to support your body's natural healing processes and enhance your overall health and well-being.

Section 7

Breathing Techniques for Specific Conditions

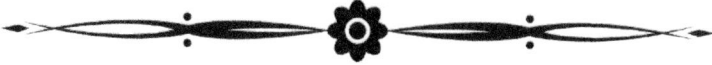

1. **Buteyko Breathing**

   a) Description: Buteyko Breathing is a technique developed by Ukrainian physician Dr. Konstantin Buteyko to help manage asthma and other respiratory conditions. This method focuses on nasal breathing, reducing breath volume, and increasing carbon dioxide levels in the blood to improve overall respiratory function.

   b) Instructions: Sit in a comfortable position with your back straight. Close your mouth and breathe gently through your nose, focusing on taking smaller, shallower breaths than usual. Try to maintain a relaxed and calm state while practicing this technique. Gradually increase the duration of your practice as you become more comfortable with the technique. Consult with a qualified Buteyko practitioner for personalized guidance and specific exercises tailored to your condition.

2. **Pursed Lip Breathing**

   a) Description: Pursed lip breathing is a technique often recommended for people with chronic obstructive pulmonary disease (COPD) or other respiratory conditions. It involves exhaling through pursed lips to create resistance, which helps to slow down the breath and improve lung function.

b) Instructions: Sit or stand in a comfortable position with your back straight. Inhale slowly through your nose for a count of two. Purse your lips as if you were about to whistle or blow out a candle. Exhale slowly through your pursed lips for a count of four. Continue to practice pursed lip breathing for several minutes, gradually increasing the duration as you become more comfortable with the technique.

3. **Breath Counting**

a) Description: Breath counting is a simple meditation technique that involves counting your breaths to help manage anxiety, stress, or other emotional disturbances. This practice helps to focus the mind and cultivate mindfulness, which can have a calming effect on the nervous system.

b) Instructions: Sit in a comfortable position with your back straight. Close your eyes and take a few deep, cleansing breaths. Begin to inhale slowly through your nose and exhale through your mouth or nose, counting "one" silently to yourself as you exhale. Continue to inhale and exhale, counting each exhalation until you reach the count of five. Once you reach five, start again at one. If your mind begins to wander or you lose count, gently bring your focus back to your breath and start again at one. Practice for several minutes, gradually increasing the duration as you become more comfortable with the technique.

4. **Breath Holding**

a) Description: Breath holding is a technique that involves holding your breath for short periods to help manage panic attacks or acute anxiety. This practice helps to stimulate the vagus nerve, which can have a calming effect on the nervous system and reduce feelings of anxiety.

b) Instructions: Sit or stand in a comfortable position with your back straight. Inhale slowly through your nose, then hold your breath for a count of five. Exhale slowly through your mouth or nose. Repeat this cycle several times or as needed to help manage feelings of panic or anxiety.

By incorporating these breathing techniques into your daily routine or using them as needed, you can support your body's natural healing processes and manage various health conditions. Remember to consult with your healthcare provider before beginning any new breathwork practice, especially if you have a pre-existing medical condition.

In the final section of this book, we will provide guidance on creating a personalized daily breathing practice that incorporates various techniques to meet your unique needs and goals. Through consistent practice, you can harness the transformative power of the breath to enhance your overall health and well-being.

Chapter 7

Creating a Personalized Daily Breathing Practice

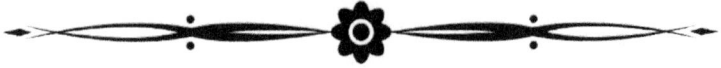

---

1. Assess Your Needs and Goals

a) Before creating your daily breathing practice, take some time to reflect on your specific needs and goals. Consider any physical, mental, or emotional challenges you may be facing, as well as your overall well-being and lifestyle.

b) Identify the breathing techniques that align with your needs and goals. For example, if you are looking to improve focus and mental clarity, you might choose to incorporate alternate nostril breathing or breath counting into your practice.

2. Experiment and Customize

a) Begin by trying the different techniques you have identified as potentially beneficial for your needs and goals. Practice each technique consistently for several days or weeks to determine its effectiveness and suitability for your daily practice.

b) Customize your practice by combining different techniques or adjusting the duration and intensity of your practice as needed. Remember that your breathwork practice should be flexible and adaptable to your changing needs and circumstances.

3. **Establish a Routine**

   a) Establishing a consistent daily routine is key to reaping the benefits of your breathing practice. Choose a specific time of day and a dedicated space to practice, and aim to maintain this routine as consistently as possible.

   b) If you find it challenging to maintain a daily practice, try incorporating shorter sessions throughout your day or practicing for shorter durations. The key is consistency and commitment.

4. **Track Your Progress**

   a) Keep a journal or log of your daily breathwork practice, noting the techniques you have practiced, the duration, and any observations or insights you may have experienced.

   b) Tracking your progress can help you identify patterns and trends, as well as highlight areas for growth and improvement.

5. **Seek Support and Guidance**

   a) Consider seeking support and guidance from a qualified breathwork practitioner, teacher, or mentor to help you deepen your practice and address any challenges or questions you may have.

   b) Engaging with a community of like-minded individuals can also provide encouragement, motivation, and inspiration for your breathwork journey.

By following these steps and incorporating the techniques and principles outlined in this book, you can create a personalized daily breathing practice that supports your unique needs and goals. Through consistent practice, you will unlock the transformative power of the breath, enhancing your overall health, focus, and well-being.

As you continue to explore the world of conscious breathing, remember that your breath is a powerful tool that can be harnessed to cultivate health, balance, and harmony in your life. May your journey with breathwork be a rewarding and transformative experience, leading you to a greater understanding of the power that lies within each inhalation and exhalation.

Chapter 8

The Benefits of Combining Different Breathing Techniques for Holistic Health and Well-being

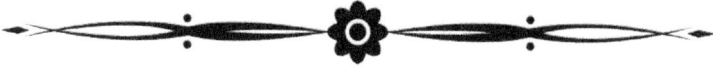

Breathing is a fundamental aspect of our existence, and there are numerous breathing techniques that can help us improve our physical, mental, and emotional health. However, combining different breathing techniques can lead to even greater benefits, as each technique has its unique advantages that can complement each other.

Here are some of the benefits of combining different breathing techniques:

1. **Enhances overall well-being**: Different breathing techniques have different effects on the body, such as calming or energizing, and combining them can lead to an overall sense of balance and well-being.

2. **Increases lung capacity**: Different techniques work on different parts of the lungs, and combining them can help expand the lung capacity and improve respiratory health.

3. **Boosts energy and focus**: Certain techniques, such as kapalabhati or bellows breath, are energizing and can help improve focus and concentration when combined with other calming techniques.

4. **Reduces stress and anxiety**: Combining calming techniques, such as diaphragmatic breathing or alternate nostril breathing, can help reduce stress and anxiety and promote relaxation.

5. **Improves digestion**: Techniques such as ujjayi and nadi shodhana have been found to improve digestion, and when combined with others, can lead to a more significant impact on digestive health.

6. **Enhances sleep quality**: Techniques such as 4-7-8 breathing or humming bee breath can help promote relaxation and enhance the quality of sleep when combined with other calming techniques.

7. **Boosts immunity**: Research has shown that certain breathing techniques, such as the Wim Hof method, can help boost the immune system, and when combined with other techniques, can lead to a more significant impact on immune health.

When combining different breathing techniques, it's essential to understand which techniques complement each other and how to integrate them into regular practice. It's also crucial to listen to the body and adjust the practice as necessary to avoid any adverse effects.

In conclusion, combining different breathing techniques can lead to a more holistic approach to health and well-being. By understanding the unique benefits of each technique and how they can complement each other, we can create a personalized practice that supports our overall health and vitality.

Chapter 9

Roles of The Role of Breathwork in Various Aspects of Life

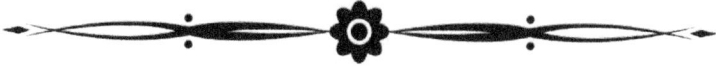

1. The Role of Breathwork in Various Spiritual Practices

Breathwork has been an integral part of various spiritual practices for centuries. Many ancient cultures, such as the Hindu, Buddhist, and Taoist traditions, have emphasized the importance of breath control in achieving spiritual growth and inner peace. In recent times, breathwork has become increasingly popular in Western spiritual practices, such as meditation and yoga.

Meditation is a practice that involves training the mind to focus and achieve a state of inner calm and clarity. Breathwork plays a vital role in meditation, as it helps to quiet the mind and create a sense of inner stillness. By focusing on the breath, practitioners can bring their attention to the present moment, letting go of thoughts and distractions that might arise.

Yoga is another spiritual practice that places great importance on breathwork. In yoga, the breath is considered the link between the mind and body. Practitioners use specific breathing techniques, such as ujjayi and pranayama, to deepen their awareness and control of the breath. These techniques help to calm the mind and relax the body, creating a sense of harmony and balance.

Breathwork is also a common practice in various forms of energy work and spiritual healing. For example, in Reiki, practitioners use breathwork to help channel energy through the body and facilitate healing. In shamanic practices, breathwork is often used to enter into altered states of consciousness and connect with the spirit world.

Overall, breathwork plays a crucial role in various spiritual practices, helping to quiet the mind, deepen awareness, and connect with a higher power. By incorporating breathwork into our spiritual practices, we can enhance our overall sense of well-being and move closer to our spiritual goals.

2. The Connection between Breath and Emotions

Breath is not only a physical process but also an emotional one. Our breath is intricately connected to our emotional states, and we can use breathwork to regulate and improve our emotional well-being. In this section, we will explore the connection between breath and emotions and how breathwork can be used as a tool for emotional regulation.

The Connection between Breath and Emotions: Breath and emotions are intimately connected. When we are anxious, stressed, or afraid, our breath becomes shallow and rapid, and we may even hold our breath. Conversely, when we are calm and relaxed, our breath is slow and deep. This connection between breath and emotions has been recognized by many spiritual traditions, including yoga and meditation.

Breathwork for Emotional Regulation: Breathwork can be used as a powerful tool for emotional regulation. By controlling our breath, we can calm our nervous system and reduce feelings of anxiety and stress. One technique that is particularly effective for emotional regulation is deep breathing. When we take slow, deep breaths, we activate the parasympathetic nervous system, which is responsible for the "rest and digest" response in our body. This can help us feel calmer and more relaxed.

Another breathwork technique that can be helpful for emotional regulation is alternate nostril breathing. This technique involves alternating the flow of breath through each nostril while using specific hand positions. Alternate nostril breathing has been shown to reduce feelings of anxiety and depression and improve overall emotional well-being.

Breathwork and Mindfulness: Breathwork can also be used as a tool for mindfulness, which is the practice of being present and fully engaged in the current moment. When we focus on our breath, we bring our attention to the present moment and become more aware of our thoughts and feelings. This can help us develop a greater sense of self-awareness and improve our emotional regulation skills.

Conclusion: Breathwork can be a powerful tool for emotional regulation and improving overall emotional well-being. By controlling our breath and practicing mindfulness, we can calm our nervous system, reduce feelings of anxiety and stress, and develop a greater sense of self-awareness. Incorporating breathwork into our daily routine can have profound effects on our emotional health and well-being.

3.Breath and the Nervous System

The nervous system is a complex network that controls and coordinates all the functions of the body, including breathing. The autonomic nervous system (ANS) is responsible for regulating the unconscious functions of the body, such as heart rate, digestion, and breathing. It is divided into two branches: the sympathetic nervous system (SNS), which activates the "fight or flight" response, and the parasympathetic nervous system (PNS), which activates the "rest and digest" response.

Breathing is a unique bodily function because it can be both voluntary and involuntary. We can consciously control our breathing, but most of the time, it happens automatically. The way we breathe can affect the balance between the SNS and PNS, and thus influence our overall state of arousal.

Studies have shown that certain breathing techniques can activate the PNS and help reduce stress and anxiety. Slow, deep breathing, for example, has been shown to slow down the heart rate and lower blood pressure, which are markers of relaxation. This type of breathing can also help regulate the levels of carbon dioxide and oxygen in the body, which can have a calming effect on the nervous system.

Other breathing techniques, such as Kapalabhati and Bhastrika, can activate the SNS and increase energy and alertness. These techniques involve rapid, forceful breathing, which can increase oxygen uptake and stimulate the release of adrenaline and other stress hormones.

Regular practice of breathwork can help train the nervous system to respond more effectively to stressors and improve overall resilience. It can also help individuals develop a greater awareness of their bodily sensations and emotions, which can be useful in managing stress and anxiety.

Incorporating breathwork into a daily routine can be a simple and effective way to reduce stress and promote relaxation. It can also be used as a complementary therapy for individuals with anxiety disorders, PTSD, and other stress-related conditions.

In conclusion, the relationship between breath and the nervous system is a powerful one, and the practice of breathwork can have significant effects on our overall well-being. By incorporating various breathing techniques into our daily routines, we can learn to regulate our emotional and physiological states and promote optimal health and resilience.

4.The Connection Between Breath and the Brain

Breathwork has been shown to have a positive impact on cognitive function and mental clarity. The connection between breath and the brain is well-established, and studies have found that certain breathing techniques can stimulate specific areas of the brain, leading to improved mental function.

One of the key benefits of breathwork on the brain is its ability to reduce stress and anxiety. When we experience stress or anxiety, our breathing patterns become shallow and rapid, which can lead to a decrease in oxygen levels in the body. This lack of oxygen can have a negative impact on the brain, leading to a decrease in cognitive function and mental clarity. By practicing deep breathing and other breathwork techniques, we can counteract this negative impact and promote a state of relaxation and calm.

Research has also shown that breathwork can improve memory and concentration. This is because deep breathing can increase blood flow and oxygen to the brain, which can improve brain function and enhance cognitive abilities.

In addition to reducing stress and improving cognitive function, breathwork can also have a positive impact on mood and emotional well-being. Certain breathing techniques, such as slow, deep breathing, have been found to increase the release of endorphins, which are the body's natural mood enhancers. This can lead to feelings of happiness, relaxation, and overall well-being.

Overall, the connection between breath and the brain is clear, and incorporating breathwork into your daily routine can have significant benefits for mental function, emotional well-being, and overall health. Whether you're looking to reduce stress and anxiety, improve cognitive function, or simply enhance your overall sense of well-being, breathwork is a powerful tool that can help you achieve your goals.

5. The Connection Between Breath and Sleep

Many of us struggle with getting enough restful sleep, and there are various factors that can contribute to this, including stress, anxiety, and poor sleep habits. However, what we may not realize is that our breathing patterns also play a significant role in the quality of our sleep.

During sleep, our bodies naturally slow down and our breathing patterns become more regular and rhythmic. This allows for the body to relax and for the brain to enter into deeper states of rest and rejuvenation. However, if our breathing is shallow or irregular during sleep, it can disrupt this natural process and lead to a less restful sleep.

One of the most common breathing issues during sleep is sleep apnea, which is a condition where breathing pauses and resumes repeatedly throughout the night. This can cause disruptions to sleep and lead to daytime fatigue, among other symptoms. Other breathing issues during sleep may include snoring or mouth breathing, which can also disrupt sleep quality.

Fortunately, there are various breathwork techniques that can help improve breathing patterns during sleep and promote a more restful sleep. Some of these techniques may include:

- Diaphragmatic breathing: This technique focuses on breathing deeply and fully from the diaphragm, which can help relax the body and promote deeper breathing patterns during sleep.

- Alternate nostril breathing: This technique involves breathing in through one nostril and out through the other, which can help balance the nervous system and promote relaxation.

- Humming bee breath: This technique involves creating a humming sound during exhalation, which can help relax the body and promote deeper breathing patterns.

- 4-7-8 breathing: This technique involves inhaling for a count of 4, holding the breath for a count of 7, and exhaling for a count of 8, which can help calm the nervous system and promote relaxation.

In addition to these techniques, there are also lifestyle changes that can improve breathing patterns during sleep, such as maintaining a regular sleep schedule, avoiding caffeine and alcohol before bedtime, and sleeping in a comfortable and supportive position.

By incorporating breathwork techniques and healthy sleep habits into our daily routines, we can improve the quality of our sleep and wake up feeling more refreshed and rejuvenated.

6. The Importance of Proper Breathing Techniques in Sports and Athletic Performance

Athletes often focus on their physical fitness, strength, and endurance to improve their performance. However, one aspect that is often overlooked is the importance of proper breathing techniques. Breathing is an essential function of the human body, and it plays a vital role in athletic performance. In this section, we will explore the connection between proper breathing techniques and sports performance.

The Role of Breathing in Sports Performance: Breathing is essential for providing oxygen to the body, which is necessary for energy production during physical activity. When we exercise, our muscles require more oxygen than when we are at rest. Proper breathing techniques can help ensure that the body is receiving the oxygen it needs to perform optimally. Additionally, proper breathing can help reduce fatigue and improve endurance, allowing athletes to perform for longer periods without tiring.

Common Breathing Techniques Used in Sports: There are several common breathing techniques that athletes use to improve their performance. These include:

1. Diaphragmatic Breathing: Also known as belly breathing, diaphragmatic breathing involves inhaling deeply through the nose, allowing the belly to expand, and exhaling through the mouth.

2. Nasal Breathing: Nasal breathing involves inhaling and exhaling through the nose. This technique can help filter and warm the air before it enters the lungs, improving oxygen uptake and reducing the risk of injury.

3. Pursed Lip Breathing: Pursed lip breathing involves exhaling through pursed lips, as if blowing out a candle. This technique can help improve breathing efficiency, reducing the risk of fatigue.

4. Interval Breathing: Interval breathing involves alternating between short, rapid breaths and slower, deeper breaths. This technique can help improve endurance and reduce fatigue.

Benefits of Proper Breathing Techniques in Sports: Proper breathing techniques can provide several benefits for athletes, including:

1. Improved Oxygen Uptake: Proper breathing techniques can help improve oxygen uptake, allowing the body to produce more energy during physical activity.

2. Reduced Fatigue: By improving oxygen uptake and reducing the buildup of carbon dioxide in the body, proper breathing techniques can help reduce fatigue, allowing athletes to perform for longer periods.

3. Improved Endurance: Proper breathing techniques can help improve endurance by reducing the need for the body to use anaerobic energy production, which can cause fatigue.

4. Reduced Risk of Injury: Proper breathing techniques, such as nasal breathing, can help warm and filter the air before it enters the lungs, reducing the risk of injury.

Conclusion: In conclusion, proper breathing techniques are an essential component of sports performance. By improving oxygen uptake, reducing fatigue, and improving endurance, athletes can benefit greatly from incorporating proper breathing techniques into their training routines.

7. History and Evolution of Breathwork Practices

Breathwork practices have been used for thousands of years in various cultures and traditions around the world. In ancient times, people understood the importance of breath for their physical, mental, and spiritual well-being. Today, many of these practices have been refined and adapted to meet the needs of modern society. This section will explore the history and evolution of breathwork practices across different cultures and traditions.

The earliest recorded breathwork practices can be traced back to ancient India, where the practice of pranayama was developed as a component of yoga. Pranayama involves various techniques of breath control, which were used to promote physical and mental health and to facilitate meditation. Pranayama techniques were later incorporated into Ayurvedic medicine, which is still widely practiced in India today.

In ancient China, the practice of qigong also incorporated breathwork techniques. Qigong is a system of exercise and meditation that focuses on the cultivation of qi, or life force energy, within the body. Qigong practitioners use a variety of breathing techniques to regulate their energy and promote health and longevity.

In Japan, the practice of Zen meditation also emphasizes the importance of breathwork. Zen meditation is a form of Buddhist meditation that focuses on mindfulness and the cultivation of inner peace. Zen practitioners use breathwork techniques to quiet the mind and achieve a state of deep relaxation.

Breathwork practices are also found in traditional African and Native American cultures. For example, the San Bushmen of the Kalahari Desert in southern Africa use a technique called "boiling the breath," which involves taking short, rapid breaths to increase energy and endurance. In Native American cultures, the use of breathwork is often associated with vision quests and other spiritual practices.

In the West, the practice of breathwork gained popularity in the 20th century with the development of various therapeutic techniques. For example, the psychotherapist Wilhelm Reich developed a technique called "deep breathing," which was used to release emotional tension and promote physical and mental health. In the 1960s and 1970s, various alternative therapies, such as rebirthing and holotropic breathwork, also incorporated breathwork techniques as a means of accessing the unconscious mind and promoting healing.

Today, breathwork practices continue to evolve and adapt to meet the needs of modern society. Many people use breathwork techniques as a means of reducing stress, improving physical health, and promoting spiritual growth. Breathwork practices are also gaining recognition in the fields of medicine and sports performance, as researchers uncover the many benefits of proper breathing techniques.

Overall, the history and evolution of breathwork practices across different cultures and traditions highlight the universal importance of breath for human health and well-being. As we continue to explore and refine these techniques, we can deepen our understanding of the connection between breath, body, and mind, and tap into the many benefits that proper breathing can offer.

8. Tools and Technologies for Breathwork Practice

In addition to traditional breathwork techniques, there are a variety of tools and technologies available today that can enhance and monitor breathwork practice. These tools can help individuals deepen their practice, track progress, and optimize their breathing for various health and performance goals.

1. *Breathwork apps*: There are numerous apps available today that offer guided breathing exercises, including popular options like Headspace, Calm, and Breathe.

These apps can help individuals learn new techniques and develop a regular breathing practice.

2. **Breath meters**: Breath meters, such as the Co2ntrol device, allow individuals to measure their carbon dioxide levels and adjust their breathing accordingly. By tracking CO_2 levels, individuals can optimize their breathing for optimal health and performance.

3. **Biofeedback devices**: Biofeedback devices, such as heart rate variability (HRV) monitors and pulse oximeters, can provide real-time feedback on breathing patterns and help individuals learn to control their breathing for various health and performance benefits.

4. **Breathing masks**: Breathing masks, such as the O2trainer, restrict air intake and force individuals to breathe more deeply and efficiently. These masks are particularly useful for athletes looking to improve their endurance and overall performance.

5. **Breathwork workshops and retreats**: Many breathwork practitioners offer workshops and retreats where individuals can learn new techniques and deepen their practice in a supportive and immersive environment.

Incorporating these tools and technologies into a regular breathwork practice can help individuals optimize their breathing for various health and performance benefits. However, it is important to remember that these tools should be used in conjunction with traditional breathwork techniques and under the guidance of a qualified practitioner.

9. The Intersection of Breathwork and Mindfulness Practices

Breathwork and mindfulness practices have a lot in common, and incorporating both can lead to a deeper level of awareness and presence. In this section, we'll explore the connection between breathwork and mindfulness, and how breath awareness can enhance mindfulness meditation.

Mindfulness meditation involves bringing attention to the present moment with a non-judgmental and curious attitude. Breath is often used as an anchor to bring the mind back to the present when it wanders. Similarly, breathwork emphasizes focusing on the breath as a means of regulating the body and calming the mind.

One way to incorporate breathwork into mindfulness practice is through breath awareness meditation. This involves simply observing the breath without trying to change it, noticing the sensations of the breath in the body, and bringing the mind back to breath whenever it wanders. This practice can help cultivate a deeper sense of calm and relaxation.

Another way to combine breathwork and mindfulness is through body scan meditation. In this practice, attention is brought to each part of the body, noticing any sensations or tension, and using the breath to release any tightness or discomfort. This practice can be particularly helpful for reducing physical tension and increasing body awareness.

Breathwork can also enhance other mindfulness practices, such as loving-kindness meditation. By incorporating deep breathing techniques and visualization, individuals can cultivate a sense of compassion and love towards themselves and others.

Overall, incorporating breathwork into mindfulness practices can deepen awareness, reduce stress, and enhance overall well-being. By combining the two practices, individuals can tap into the full potential of their breath and mind-body connection.

10: The Role of Breathwork in Personal Growth and Transformation

Breathwork has long been known for its potential to facilitate personal growth and transformation. Practitioners of breathwork believe that by focusing on the breath and using specific techniques, they can gain a deeper understanding of themselves and their place in the world.

One way in which breathwork can facilitate personal growth is through the release of emotional blockages. By bringing awareness to the breath and using specific techniques, individuals can access and release emotions that have been held in the body. This can lead to a greater sense of emotional well-being and the ability to move forward in life with greater clarity and purpose.

Breathwork can also be a powerful tool for self-discovery. By using the breath to enter into a state of deep relaxation, individuals can gain access to their innermost thoughts and feelings. This can be especially helpful for those who are struggling with personal or professional issues, as it can help them gain clarity and perspective on their situation.

In addition to facilitating emotional release and self-discovery, breathwork can also be a tool for personal empowerment. By practicing breathwork regularly, individuals can develop a greater sense of inner strength and resilience. This can help them to better navigate the challenges of daily life and to approach difficult situations with greater confidence and ease.

One specific area in which breathwork has been found to be particularly effective is in the treatment of trauma. Research has shown that breathwork can help individuals to process and release traumatic experiences, leading to a greater sense of emotional and psychological well-being.

Overall, the potential benefits of breathwork for personal growth and transformation are vast. By incorporating breathwork into their daily routine, individuals can gain access to a deeper sense of self-awareness, emotional healing, and personal empowerment.

11. The Role of Breathwork and Finance

While the connection between breathwork and finance may not seem immediately apparent, there is a growing body of evidence to suggest that the two are more closely linked than we may realize. One way in which breathwork can impact our finances is through its potential to reduce stress and increase overall well-being. When we are stressed, our decision-making abilities can become impaired, leading to poor financial choices and potentially costly mistakes. By practicing breathwork, individuals can reduce their stress levels and improve their ability to make clear-headed decisions about their finances.

Another way in which breathwork can impact on our finances is through its potential to increase our focus and productivity. By incorporating breathwork into their daily routine, individuals can develop a greater sense of mental clarity and focus, allowing them to better tackle their work and financial goals. Additionally, by reducing distractions and increasing focus, breathwork can help individuals to be more efficient with their time, potentially leading to increased income and financial stability.

Breathwork can also be a powerful tool for cultivating abundance and prosperity. By practicing gratitude and visualization techniques during breathwork sessions, individuals can shift their mindset towards one of abundance and attract more positive financial opportunities into their lives.

Overall, the potential benefits of breathwork for financial well-being are vast. By incorporating breathwork into their daily routine, individuals can reduce stress, increase focus and productivity, and cultivate a mindset of abundance and prosperity, leading to greater financial stability and success.

Chapter 10: Case studies

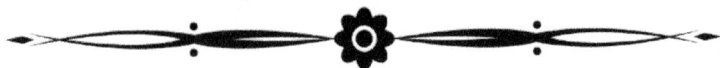

Here are some examples of case studies that could be used for different breathing techniques:

1. *Diaphragmatic breathing*: A study conducted on 40 healthy adults found that practicing diaphragmatic breathing for just 20 minutes a day for eight weeks significantly reduced stress levels and improved heart rate variability (HRV), a measure of overall heart health. Participants reported feeling more relaxed and better able to handle stressful situations after practicing diaphragmatic breathing regularly.

2. *Box breathing*: A study published in the Journal of Alternative and Complementary Medicine found that box breathing can help to reduce symptoms of post-traumatic stress disorder (PTSD). In the study, veterans with PTSD were taught box breathing and reported significant improvements in their symptoms, including reduced anxiety and sleep disturbances.

3. *Ujjayi breath*: A case study published in the International Journal of Yoga Therapy documented the use of ujjayi breath in the treatment of anxiety and depression in a 31-year-old female. After practicing ujjayi breath for six months, the patient reported significant improvements in her symptoms and was able to reduce her medication dosage.

4. *Nadi shodhana*: A study conducted on 30 university students found that practicing nadi shodhana for just 10

minutes a day for four weeks significantly improved cognitive function and attention span. Participants reported feeling more focused and mentally alert after practicing Nadi Shodhana regularly.

5. *Holotropic breathwork*: A case study published in the Journal of Transpersonal Psychology documented the use of holotropic breathwork in the treatment of chronic pain in a 58-year-old female. After several sessions of holotropic breathwork, the patient reported significant reductions in her pain levels and improved quality of life.

6. *Sitali Pranayama*: A case study published in the Journal of Ayurveda and Integrative Medicine documented the use of Sitali Pranayama in the management of hypertension in a 47-year-old male. After practicing Sitali Pranayama for three months, the patient's blood pressure levels significantly decreased, and he reported feeling more relaxed and calm.

7. *Breath of Fire*: A study published in the International Journal of Yoga Therapy found that breath of fire can help to improve lung function in individuals with chronic obstructive pulmonary disease (COPD). Participants who practiced breath of fire for eight weeks reported significant improvements in their lung function and overall quality of life.

8. *Tummo Breathing*: A case study published in the Journal of Transpersonal Research documented the use of tummo breathing in the treatment of chronic fatigue syndrome in a 33-year-old female. After practicing tummo breathing regularly for six months, the patient

reported significant improvements in her energy levels and overall well-being.

9. *Alternate Nostril Breathing*: A study published in the International Journal of Yoga Therapy found that alternate nostril breathing can help to reduce symptoms of depression and anxiety. Participants who practiced alternate nostril breathing for six weeks reported significant reductions in their symptoms and improved overall mental health.

10. *2-to-1 Breathing*: A case study published in the Journal of Clinical and Diagnostic Research documented the use of 2-to-1 breathing in the treatment of insomnia in a 40-year-old female. After practicing 2-to-1 breathing for four weeks, the patient reported significant improvements in her sleep quality and was able to reduce her medication dosage.

These case studies are just a glimpse into the potential benefits of different breathing techniques. There are many more studies and personal anecdotes that highlight the positive impact that breathing practices can have on physical, mental, and emotional well-being. From reducing stress and anxiety to improving cognitive function and enhancing athletic performance, there is a breathing technique for nearly every situation.

As you continue to explore and experiment with different techniques, we encourage you to pay attention to your body's responses and consult with a healthcare professional if you have any concerns. The possibilities for transformation through breathing practices are vast, and we hope that these case studies inspire you to further integrate these techniques into your daily life.

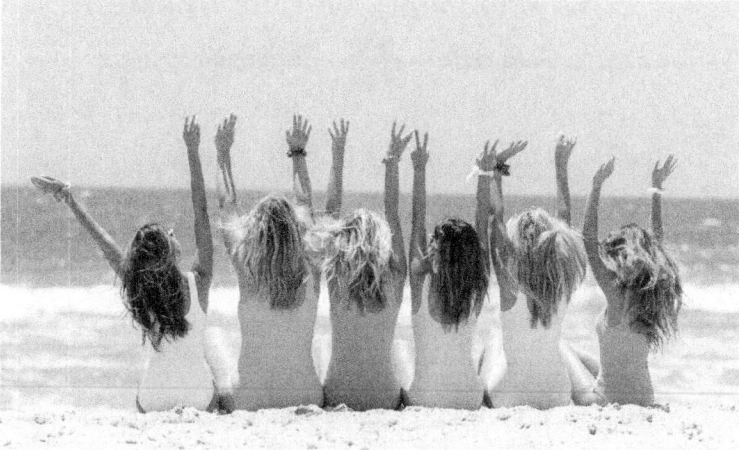

Chapter 11

Precautions and Contraindications

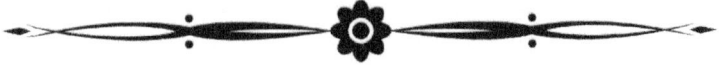

Potential Drawbacks and Risks of Breathwork

Breathwork is generally considered to be a safe and beneficial practice for most individuals. However, like any form of physical or mental exercise, there are potential risks and drawbacks to consider. In this section, we will explore some of the potential risks associated with breathwork and the precautions that individuals should take to practice safely.

1. **Hyperventilation**: One of the most common risks associated with breathwork is hyperventilation, which occurs when an individual breathes too quickly or deeply, leading to an imbalance of oxygen and carbon dioxide in the blood. This can cause symptoms such as dizziness, lightheadedness, and tingling in the extremities. To avoid hyperventilation, it is important to start slowly and gradually increase the intensity of the practice over time.

2. **Emotional release**: Breathwork has the potential to trigger intense emotional responses, which can be both cathartic and overwhelming. Individuals who have experienced trauma or have a history of emotional instability should approach breathwork with caution and seek the guidance of a qualified practitioner.

3. **Pre-existing health conditions**: Individuals with pre-existing health conditions such as asthma, chronic obstructive pulmonary disease (COPD), or cardiovascular disease should consult with a healthcare provider before practicing breathwork, as certain techniques may not be suitable for their condition.

4. **Spiritual bypassing**: Some individuals may use breathwork as a means of avoiding or bypassing deeper emotional or psychological issues, which can lead to a false sense of healing or spiritual bypassing. It is important to approach breathwork as a complementary practice to other forms of therapy or personal growth work.

To practice breathwork safely and effectively, it is important to seek the guidance of a qualified practitioner and to approach the practice with patience and self-awareness. It is also important to honor any physical or emotional limitations and to listen to the body's signals during practice. By taking these precautions, individuals can reap the many benefits of breathwork while minimizing the potential risks.

1. **General Safety Guidelines**

   a) Always approach breathwork with a sense of curiosity and respect for your body's limits. b. Practice in a safe and comfortable environment, free of distractions and potential hazards.

   b) If at any point you feel lightheaded, dizzy, or experience discomfort, stop practicing and return to normal breathing.

2. Potential Risks and Contraindications for Each Technique

a) While most breathing techniques are safe for the general population, some may carry potential risks or contraindications for individuals with specific health conditions.

b) Always read and follow the precautions and contraindications provided for each technique, and consult with a healthcare professional if you are unsure about the suitability of a particular practice for your circumstances.

3. Consulting with Healthcare Professionals When Needed

a) If you have pre-existing health conditions, are pregnant, or are taking medication, consult with a healthcare professional before starting any breathwork practice.

b) If you experience any adverse effects or worsening symptoms while practicing breathwork, seek professional advice immediately.

Chapter 12: Additional Research

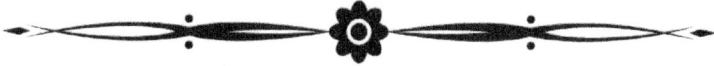

1. **Apps and Technology for Practicing Breathing Techniques**
   a) There are numerous apps and devices available to support your breathwork practice, such as guided meditation apps, breath pacer apps, and wearable devices that monitor your breathing patterns.

   b) Some popular apps include Calm, Headspace, Breathe+, and Prana Breath.

2. **Further Reading and Research**
   a) Books such as "The Oxygen Advantage" by Patrick McKeown, "Breath: The New Science of a Lost Art" by James Nestor, and "The Healing Power of the Breath" by Dr. Richard Brown and Dr. Patricia Gerbarg offer in-depth information and additional techniques.

   b) Online resources, such as YouTube channels, blogs, and websites dedicated to breathwork, can provide further guidance and inspiration.

   c) Diaphragmatic breathing: A study published in the Journal of Thoracic Disease found that diaphragmatic breathing can improve lung function and reduce respiratory distress in patients with chronic obstructive pulmonary disease (COPD) (https://www.ncbi.nlm.nih.gov/pmc/articles/PMC738856 5/). Another study published in the Journal of Clinical Nursing found that diaphragmatic breathing can reduce anxiety and improve sleep quality in patients with type 2 diabetes (https://pubmed.ncbi.nlm.nih.gov/33107455/).

d) Zen breathing: A study published in the Journal of Alternative and Complementary Medicine found that Zen breathing can improve mood and reduce symptoms of anxiety and depression in college students (https://pubmed.ncbi.nlm.nih.gov/23607839/).

e) Resonant breathing: A study published in the International Journal of Behavioral Medicine found that resonant breathing can improve heart rate variability and reduce symptoms of anxiety and depression in patients with post-traumatic stress disorder (PTSD) (https://pubmed.ncbi.nlm.nih.gov/30269221/).

f) Alternate nostril breathing: A study published in the International Journal of Yoga Therapy found that alternate nostril breathing can improve attention and cognitive performance in healthy adults (https://www.ncbi.nlm.nih.gov/pmc/articles/PMC5545948/).

g) Breath of fire: A case study published in the International Journal of Yoga Therapy found that breath of fire can reduce symptoms of depression and anxiety in a patient with a history of childhood trauma (https://www.ncbi.nlm.nih.gov/pmc/articles/PMC6235834/).

h) Wim Hof method: A case study published in the Journal of Psychopharmacology found that the Wim Hof method can reduce symptoms of depression and anxiety in a patient with treatment-resistant depression (https://pubmed.ncbi.nlm.nih.gov/30081784/).

i) Holotropic breathwork: A study published in the Journal of Transpersonal Psychology found that holotropic breathwork can reduce symptoms of anxiety and depression in adults with a history of childhood trauma (https://www.jstor.org/stable/23266839).

It's important to note that case studies and research studies may not be applicable to everyone and should not be seen as a replacement for professional medical advice. Resources and citations for these studies can be included in the book's references section.

3. **Workshops and Courses on Breathwork**
   a) Attending workshops, classes, or retreats led by experienced breathwork practitioners can deepen your understanding and practice.

   b) Online courses and webinars are also available for those who prefer to learn from the comfort of their own home.

CONCLUSION

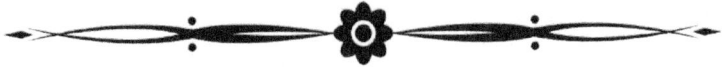

In conclusion, developing breathwork practice can be a powerful tool for personal growth and transformation. Through conscious breathing, we can regulate our physical, mental, and emotional states, and tap into the innate wisdom and healing capacity of our bodies. The techniques presented in this guide offer a diverse range of approaches to breathwork, each with its own benefits and applications. Whether you choose to focus on a few techniques or explore them all, the journey of breath awareness and practice is a lifelong one that can offer new insights and discoveries at every turn.

As you continue to deepen your understanding and connection with your breath, I encourage you to approach your practice with an open mind and heart, and to be patient and compassionate with yourself along the way. It's natural to encounter challenges or setbacks in any practice, but with dedication and perseverance, you can cultivate a more profound and fulfilling relationship with your breath. Remember to always listen to your body and to seek guidance from a qualified practitioner if you have any concerns or questions about your practice.

Finally, I hope this guide has provided you with a solid foundation and inspiration for your breathwork journey. There are many resources available for further exploration and study, from books and online courses to workshops and retreats. I wish you all the best in your continued exploration of the vast and wondrous world of conscious breathing.

THANK YOU

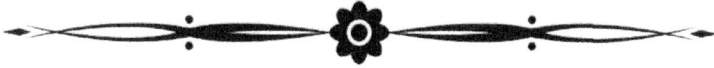

Thank you for reading this book on the power of breath and conscious breathing. We hope that it has provided you with valuable insights, techniques, and inspiration for your own breathwork practice.

We would like to express our gratitude to all the teachers, practitioners, researchers, and authors who have contributed to the field of breathwork and helped to make this book possible. Your dedication, wisdom, and generosity have been instrumental in shaping the way we understand and approach breathwork today.

We would also like to thank our families, friends, and colleagues for their support, encouragement, and patience throughout the writing and publishing process. Your love and understanding have been a constant source of inspiration and motivation.

Finally, we extend our gratitude to you, the reader, for your interest, curiosity, and willingness to explore the world of conscious breathing. We hope that this book has sparked your passion for breathwork and that it will continue to guide and inspire you on your journey of self-discovery and transformation.

Thank you, and may you always breathe deeply, fully, and consciously.

Breathe
By Melody Wallack

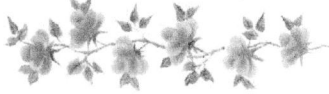

Breathe deep, inhale life's sweet air
Let go of worries, release all care
Feel the rise and fall of your chest
Each breath a gift, a moment blessed
***

With every inhale, a chance to renew
And with each exhale, let go of what no longer serves you
The breath is a guide, a path to find
A connection to self, a peace of mind
***

So take a moment, and just breathe
Let the rhythm of your breath relieve
The stress and tension of the day
As you breathe, let worries fade away
***

Inhale, exhale, a simple act
Yet it has the power to impact
Your mind, your body, your very soul
Breathe in the present, and let yourself feel whole
***

Breathe in love, breathe out fear
Let your breath guide you, and draw near
To the present moment, where all is well
Breathe deep, and let your worries quell.

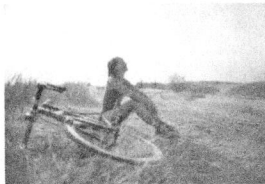

Printed in Great Britain
by Amazon